The Anti-Burnout Book

How to avoid burning out and your recovery toolkit if you do

Dr Emma Hepburn

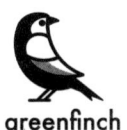
greenfinch

Praise for *The Anti-Burnout Book*

'The anti-burnout rebellion we all need to join. This book will help you break free from living like a zombie with burnout and find your fire.' – **Dr Martha Deiros Collado, bestselling author and clinical psychologist**

'Essential reading for anyone who wants to understand and recover from burnout. In this honest, practical, and deeply compassionate guide, Emma brings clarity to the complex experience of burnout and offers tools that genuinely help. And when reading feels too much, her beautiful illustrations tell you everything you need to know.' – **Dr Julie Smith, clinical psychologist and million-copy bestselling author**

'This book is a lifeline. It's wise, warm and wonderfully practical – the hand you need to hold when you're running on empty. Dr Emma doesn't just explain burnout; she gently walks you out of it. It will quite literally change the way you live.' – **Holly Tucker MBE**

'*The Anti-Burnout Book* is a manual for rebuilding your energy, your boundaries, and your belief that you're worth caring for.
Every leader, every parent, every carer, every woman needs this.'
– **Lauren Currie, Founder and CEO UPFRONT**

'A deeply human guide to protect yourself from burnout and the accessible toolkit you need to reclaim your vitality and joy. Reassuring and compassionate, Emma is the voice you need to expedite healing. The only book on burnout you need.' - **Suzy Reading, psychologist and author**

'*The Anti-Burnout Book* is clinically robust and deeply compassionate. Emma brings clarity to an experience that so often feels chaotic and shame-filled, grounding psychological insight in her own lived experience so the book feels human, relatable and trustworthy. I'll be recommending often.' – **Dr Emma Svanberg, clinical psychologist**

Contents

Introduction   1

Part 1: Getting to Know Burnout

1   What is burnout? And how do I know it's happened?   14
2   Building a burnout tree: Understanding what contributes to burnout   36

Part 2: How to Avoid Burnout

3   Under pressure: Stress, stress and more stress   62
4   Beliefs and burnout   85
5   Let's get physical, and emotional   106
6   Making work work for you: Let's take a look at your day job   120
7   Who cares? Caring and the other roles in our lives   144
8   Different brains and burnout: Why burnout is a neurodiversity issue   166

Part 3: Relighting Your Fire: What To Do If You Are Burned Out

9   The emotional impact of burnout   190
10   The physical impact of burnout   212
11   Piecing your life back together after burnout   235
12   Building back stronger   262

Conclusion   289
Notes   291
Further Reading   306
Index   309

Introduction

I burned out. Despite being a clinical psychologist for over twenty years and knowing all the tricks and tools to identify and manage stress, I burned out. Despite writing books on how to support wellbeing, I burned out. Despite working in a job that I love, which fits with my values, I burned out. Despite feeling very lucky about my life, I burned out.

If that feels like a confessional, that's because it's exactly how it felt to me. I had to confess I was burned out. I had to admit to myself it wasn't something that just happened to other people, it was something happening to me. Now, of course I didn't think I was immune to mental or physical health difficulties. I knew from research and working with lots of patients that we all have ups and downs and that most people struggle at some point in their life. In fact, research indicates that staying mentally well throughout your life is rarer than experiencing poor mental health at some point.[1] I strongly advocate that given the right (or wrong) mix of person and environment, we are all susceptible to poor mental health or just feeling totally rubbish for a longer period than we might normally.

However, I mistakenly thought that, as a clinical psychologist I had the skills to effectively manage stress, be able to spot signs early and take action – even if that meant seeking professional help. But as my realization dawned, I had to admit

The Anti-Burnout Book

I was chronically burned out and had only noticed when I was in the pits of it. This moment of realization occurred with a big sprinkling of irony.

So, what happened?

During the Covid-19 pandemic I moved from a clinical role in neuropsychology (working with brain injuries) to lead a workplace team, which aimed to improve wellbeing in a healthcare organization. I considered this a challenging but important role, as caring professionals have always been more susceptible to poor mental health and burnout compared to the general population (and the pandemic exacerbated this risk). As part of this work I supported individual staff members who shared their difficult and traumatic experiences working on the front line. To be honest, I felt lucky to work in this role and hear these things, rather than have the direct experiences these people had gone through.

What became abundantly clear through these stories is that to support wellbeing and stop burnout proactively, we needed to work not just with individuals but also target the environments in which they work. Our aims as a staff wellbeing service were to support people to stay well and to intervene early, not just to respond when things had already gone wrong. And there is the first sprinkling of irony – clearly, I didn't manage to apply this to myself.

To support our aims, we designed and sent out several wellbeing surveys to staff – and a large number of my colleagues said they felt exhausted and burned out. I decided to take the survey myself. I admit this was partly to boost numbers to meet our target, but nevertheless I filled it out as honestly as I could. Like any good psychologist, I debated

Introduction

my answers to most of the questions. However, one question elicited an uncharacteristically definitive response: Do you feel too tired after work to do the things you enjoy? I answered with immediate certainty: Always.

But, ironically, this wasn't my moment of realization, although it should have been. And this wasn't a single point of failure – I missed multiple indicators that I was becoming burned out.

Ignoring the signs

Humans are meaning-making creatures. However, sometimes we find explanations of what's going on that are removed from the overall picture, which prevents us from piecing together the big picture. The crippling tiredness? Well, a large proportion of the workplace was telling me they felt this way, so it was clearly just a normal reaction to pandemic conditions. The extra effort I was putting in to achieve my normal level of work? I just needed to work harder. The rash rising from my ear? Must just be the masks rubbing that I had to wear every day. The thinning hair? Clearly it was due to the number of showers I was taking when returning home from the hospital, to try to ensure the virus didn't creep into my family home. The inevitable shutter that came down in my brain midway through the day, making my speech slur and normal cognitive functioning impossible? Hmm, I suppose I should really see my doctor about that. These disparate pieces were clearly part of a bigger puzzle, but they did not join up in my (to be fair, totally exhausted and not thinking clearly) mind.

There was something else at play here too – we tend to be dismissive and invalidating of our own experiences. I've seen this thousands of times in people I have worked with and friends and family. We minimize our own experiences and emotions as something inconsequential that we should just shrug off. But surely I shouldn't have been guilty of this – I mean, I'm a clinical psychologist who writes books on noticing and validating our emotions. Come on, if anyone should be able to validate their experiences, it should be me! Working with people who had been through traumatic and life-changing events made me focus on what I did have. I told myself I am lucky, other people have it much worse. This outlook on life has been predominantly helpful to me, but during burnout it gradually transformed into a subtle dismissiveness that meant I minimized what was happening and saw it as 'not that bad'.

In hindsight, it's clear what was happening. Clinical psychologists understand people's difficulties by co-creating a formulation with them. A formulation gives a full picture: it makes sense of someone's experiences, puts them in context; it helps us to understand the factors that contributed to their development, what's exacerbating and what's helping; and indicates what to do next to help overcome the difficulties.

It's not hard to write a formulation of what happened to me: the causal factors were glaringly obvious, in hindsight at least. So obvious that surely I should have seen it coming (shame says: 'You're a psychologist – of *all* people you should not have let this happen'). But when you're surviving day to day, with a brain that needs to make extra effort to function, the ability to reflect, notice and take the necessary action just doesn't happen. In fact, your brain is so focused on getting through the next moment or thing that it has no capacity left to focus on the wider picture or what you need to do. Until, that is, it has no choice.

Introduction

The tipping point

My moment of realization wasn't pretty, but it was necessary. It happened on what should have been a lovely weekend away in Edinburgh with two of my closest and longest friends, but instead became a point in time that smacked me in the face and ultimately shifted where I went next. I remember debating if I should go in the first place. If I'm honest, I really wanted to avoid going, not because I didn't want to see my friends but because I was so damn tired that I wasn't sure I would manage to function and speak beyond late afternoon and thought I would be rubbish company. But my husband persuaded me that I needed to see my friends and have some downtime. So, I dutifully caught the train to the beautiful city of Edinburgh, unaware that a not-so-beautiful experience was about to occur.

On the second evening, as we sat having drinks and conversation, an innocuous comment, which would, at other times, have sparked an interesting and topical conversation, tipped me over the edge. My capacity was already low and the late drinks the night before had used up every remaining ounce of energy, so I had no capacity to function beyond the mundane. It took only a tiny thing to make me overflow, like a bursting dam. In uncharacteristic behaviour, I silently left the room, leaving my friends aghast and confused, wondering what the heck I was doing. I was bemused and had no idea what I was doing either. I was in some bizarre burned-out, zombie-style autopilot, functioning (just) but with very little awareness, and my body wasn't about to let me ignore the signs any longer.

As I sat down, I started shaking violently and had a multitude of physical reactions that ranged from bizarre to scary. It was a shock reaction, with nothing ostensible at which to be shocked. My body had been running on empty for so long, with so little capacity or resources, that the additional effort of the weekend meant I was hanging on by a thread, and a frayed thread at that. It just took a teeny tiny inane thing to push my body over the edge. My friends looked after me as I shook for what felt like several hours then collapsed, exhausted, into bed. As a typical Scot, not known for demonstrative big emotions or reactions, it was far more dramatic than I would ever want to be and I woke up feeling embarrassed and ashamed (although look out for beliefs about being dramatic, as these can be problematic – more about that later). In fact, I still feel some shame and guilt about the impact of my reaction. But it was the tipping point that broke through the fugue I had been in, and on the train journey home I started putting the puzzle pieces together and saw that action was necessary.

Why I wrote this book

And that's the story of where this book came from. The nugget of an idea formed as I noticed the Emma Zombie I had become and started to speak to people about my experiences. I already knew from my work that many people in caring jobs were exhausted, but I wasn't prepared for the outpouring of exhaustion that came my way from all angles. Only a few short weeks after my disastrous trip, I returned to Edinburgh for a wellbeing festival where I spoke to other authors. Among them was Emma Gannon, who shared pieces of her own story of burnout with me and how she was managing this (she has since shared this on her Substack page and in her books[2]). As my interest was piqued, I began to notice more and more stories about exhausted people, from Katherine May in her book *Wintering*,[3] to interviews with celebrities like Beyoncé (see page 18) and Gwyneth Paltrow and athletes such as swimmer

Introduction

Tom Dean and gymnast Simone Biles. I didn't have to look hard to find stories about burnout.

In early 2023 I posted on my Instagram page that I was exhausted, predominantly to explain why I hadn't done much on there (I had been posting lots of psychology illustrations during the early pandemic as @thepsychologymum but then went quiet). I asked who else was exhausted. Although not a scientific study, the numbers were shocking: 83 per cent told me they had burned out as some point during the pandemic and 63 per cent told me they were still burned out. I asked again in 2024 and the number was even higher: 94 per cent told me they had burned out at some point since 2020. In a strange coincidence, on exactly the same day Jacinda Ardern resigned as New Zealand's prime minister, saying she no longer had enough in the tank to do the job justice. As a result, burnout hit the national headlines. It felt like my eyes were opened, and I started seeing it everywhere. Everyone was speaking about their exhaustion – and not just caring professionals: comedians, actors, singers, business people, politicians, royals, authors, publishers, students, artists, academics, mothers, carers, school kids. Anybody and everybody, regardless of profession or lifestyle, was describing exhaustion.

The stats told a similar story. High rates of burnout have been demonstrated in nearly every profession or group where it has been measured.[4] In a recent Deloitte survey, 84 per cent of millennials reported experiencing burnout in their current job, compared to 77 per cent of all respondents.[5] A 2022 report showed 66 per cent of US working parents met the criteria for burnout.[6] The pandemic had clearly taken its toll, and the whole world seemed exhausted as a result. But when people spoke about the factors contributing to their exhaustion, the pandemic was always, if anything, just part of the story, and I wondered what else was going on.

When I said I was thinking about writing a book about burnout, exhausted people used their last ounce of energy to wearily push open their rusty floodgates and share a deluge of burnout stories. The almost unanimous stock response was, 'Oh, I could speak to you about my experiences for your book.' What was going on? Which aspects of modern life were making it difficult to switch off and were creating this mass exhaustion? I was clearly not alone. My experience appeared to reflect the grand collective experience of the age, and the shape of this book emerged: an exploration of this common phenomenon, combining my experience with our collective experience, to produce an anti-burnout manifesto.

However, I was too exhausted and burned out to write. So that's where this book stayed for a while, on the shelf as an idea that I had no energy to develop into anything more. I had written three books in three years, and this, along with my other roles, had led to the point of complete exhaustion and burnout that I was at. I decided I had to 'be more Jacinda Ardern'. I needed to stop doing things I no longer had energy in the tank to do and take time to recover and rebuild my energy stores so I would be able to write again – and function in all the other roles I had, including mum, friend, wife, daughter, clinical psychologist, lecturer, manager, colleague. So the publication of this book was delayed until I was out the other side and recovered.

Through this time, my non-functioning brain would often travel to a dream world of its own, a world of no demands or pressures. I would have loved to just stop, get away from it all and rest.

Introduction

It was a fantasy to take a holiday by myself somewhere sunny, with no devices and without having to speak to anyone for an extended period of time. But, hey, people need money, children need parents, and there are all sorts of other ties. While this solution may be possible for a small group of people, it's not a choice for most. So, the solo-holiday option stayed firmly in fantasy land. Unfortunately for them, my family and friends were stuck with me (well, it was more like they stuck *with* me because I hardly ever responded to messages or phone calls during this time – sorry!) and my poorly functioning brain and body.

The idea for this book sat on the idea shelf for years while I did what was in my control to recover from burnout and regain the energy, will and enthusiasm to re-engage with life and the reality of writing. And here we are.

The road to recovery

Am I fully recovered? No, I'm left with a legacy of burnout. Physically, I still have times of complete exhaustion, the days I feel like my brain cells are churning through a murky swamp. The shutter comes down now and again and my ability to function stops. But these are rare exceptions rather than the norm and I notice, understand and respond to them. Even better, I can do something about them and rest really helps.

While formerly I felt like a shrivelled burned-out chip that had been forgotten, left in the oven and didn't resemble its original state, psychologically I do feel like me again. My enthusiasm has returned, accompanied with my (I think) healthy dose of cynicism. I'm still cautious about taking on new things but no longer dread doing anything new. My brain's ability to plan and look forward to things has returned. I no longer feel a failure at many roles in my life because I'm too exhausted to parent, friend or daughter in the way I would like. Actually, it feels cheesy and clichéd to say, but some things are better. I can't bring myself to say I have grown as a person, it's just too un-me. But I've designed my life better to protect against burnout. I am more able to align my lifestyle with my values and say no to things that don't. I have broken down old habits that didn't serve me and built ones that do. Yes, good things may have come from it, but I would rather not have burned out. I would also rather you did not burn out. In fact, I would say I am very anti-burnout.

Starting the anti-burnout rebellion

And that's where this book comes in. I truly believe we should all be anti-burnout by putting things in place, when we can, to stop us burning to a crisp. This is about looking after ourselves, of course, but it's also about understanding the systemic, cultural and contextual factors that contribute to burnout. In fact, I think we should start a rebellion because I also believe we should take action to tackle the contextual factors that lead us to burnout and build systems and cultures that are anti-burnout (workplace leaders and managers, I'm looking at you for starters). And if we can't avoid becoming that burned crisp of a chip (because we can't always control what life throws at us), we need to have the skills to rekindle and reignite our fire. We need to use our experiences to build back better and design our future lives to keep our flames burning and protect them from burning out again. So, here's my anti-burnout manifesto. I hope you enjoy it and can use it to keep your fire burning in this complex and sometimes difficult world in which we live.

Introduction

This book is set out in a way that I hope makes it as useable as possible. When I was burned out, I found books difficult to read – text swam before my eyes and too much information made me stop reading. Yes, there are some bits of my experience, and other people's too, to bring the theory to life. I share how burnout impacted me and the factors that contributed to it. But this book is not about me: it is about the research around burnout and the collective experience of it. Most importantly, this book is about you. Each of us brings unique factors to the mix. To become anti-burnout we need to understand our own mixture of person and context, how this contributes to burnout and where to take action to protect or reignite our flames.

We'll look at defining burnout, its impact and causes (both individual and contextual) and what we can do to help (before it happens and if it does). In each section there are reflection points (which you are guided through by Brian the Brain*) to think about your own experiences, and tools for understanding your situation better and supporting you on your journey. And when you have completed this book, you will become a fully-fledged founding member of the anti-burnout gang.

I firmly believe we all need to be anti-burnout, to prevent it controlling our lives or defining our modern age. I am so pleased you have joined me on this journey, so you can be anti-burnout in your own life too. Let's begin.

---

* Brian the Brain is my cartoon character, which is both the name I call my own brain and a visual representation I use in illustrations to explain how brains function and how this can contribute to difficulties, including burnout.

PART 1
Getting to Know Burnout

Chapter 1

What is burnout? And how do I know it's happened?

If I was to define burnout in my own words, I would say it is the zombification of your brain, your body and you as person as a result of work-related (and we need to think very carefully about how we define 'work') chronic stress. As a zombie, you do not feel like a fully formed person, functioning as they ought to. You may appear to be functioning to the outside word, but in reality you are only just managing to (sometimes) do the basics – anything beyond that and higher-level thought feel impossible. Exhaustion pervades every cell and dulls all your senses, yet, because your zombified brain is constantly looking out for danger, you are also always on high alert and can't switch off. Ever. Even when you sleep (that's if you even manage to sleep). You have lost the person you were and have turned into the zombie version of yourself, stumbling through life with a semi-functioning brain, trying to just get through and survive.

Now, this is my experience. As you are a unique human being, your burnout experience will probably be a bit different. Let's start by looking at the more formal definition of burnout before thinking about how it affects you.

How do we define burnout?

My description might differ to what you find in most books (they don't usually refer to zombies, for a start) where you are more likely to come across the formal World Health Organization (WHO) definition of burnout (from their diagnostic manual ICD-11 published in 2022).[1] This was the first time burnout was fully recognized[2] in a diagnostic manual, although clearly not the first time it ever existed. References to what sounds like burnout can be found throughout historical literature from Shakespeare in the 16th century to Graham Greene in his 1960 book aptly titled *A Burnt-Out Case*. Some people even argue burnout descriptions can be found in the Bible.[3]

Burnout was first used as a clinical term in the 1970s when a psychiatrist called Freudenberger[4] recognized it as a common group of symptoms in a clinic in which he was working (if you read his obituary, it suggests he was a workaholic who also burned out).[5] Around this time, the first scientific research by Maslach and colleagues looking at burnout in social workers was also underway.[6] Since this time, research and clinical interest has grown exponentially, initially mainly in caring professions and then to other groups, until we get to the point we are at today. No doubt exacerbated by the pandemic, it now seems burnout is viewed as a modern ubiquitous phenomenon, widely discussed in media, social media, books, podcasts, interviews and general society. Burnout appears everywhere you look, and many, many people see themselves in burnout descriptions. Try this out for yourself: speak to someone about burnout and I can almost guarantee they will identify with it in some way.

Let's turn back to that formal definition. Intriguingly, WHO call burnout an occupational phenomenon **not** (and that is in bold in their description!) a medical illness – we'll come back to think about what that means later. In the 2022 WHO diagnostic manual (ICD-11) definition, burnout is described as:

> *...a syndrome conceptualized from chronic workplace stress that has not been successfully managed.*

There are a couple of points of interest here. Firstly, how do we define workplaces and work itself, because this will affect who we define as burned out. Secondly, who is not successfully managing the stress. Is it you as an individual? Or the workplace? Or both? We'll look at all these factors, but let's first dig down into the detail of how burnout is defined. Researchers Maslach and colleagues defined it with three separate but interlinked dimensions, and developed validated measures of burnout, which stipulate that all three dimensions must be present to identify someone as burned out – exhaustion alone is not enough. In line with this definition, the ICD-11 tells us burnout is characterized by symptoms in these three dimensions:

1. Feelings of energy depletion or exhaustion.
2. Increased mental distance from/negativism or cynicism related to one's job.
3. Reduced personal efficacy.

What does burnout look and feel like?

Okay, great, we have a definition. But what does that actually look and feel like in real life? As with all formal definitions, it might look slightly different for each person. While I can tell you my perspective, and pull some examples from how other people have described their burnout, this might look slightly different for you within each dimension.

Here's how burnout looked and felt for me, in relation to the defined three dimensions.

Dimension 1: Feelings of energy depletion or exhaustion

I was experiencing an exhaustion so pervasive that it leached into everything I did and affected every area of my life. It meant I had to make extra effort to complete tasks I had to do, such as work. But this used up my reserves and I had no energy left for the even more important tasks, such as being a mum. At some point during the day, I felt like a shutter came down on my brain, which meant I could no longer function. My brain was just functioning at a basic level, on zombie autopilot, and higher brain functioning wasn't possible. All abilities felt slowed down, and what used to be enjoyable, fun or easy now felt difficult.

I looked back on my former self and was in awe at how I had managed to function in daily life, let alone write a book. I was certain I would never be able to write a book again. My brain felt like the neurons had turned to soup and were no longer able to communicate, which impacted on all my cognitive functioning, including my communication - my speech became slow and slurred after the shutter came down. Physically, exercise seemed impossible as I often had to stop halfway up our (not big) stairs and steel myself to keep going. In what felt like a cruel irony, although I was exhausted, at the same time I was constantly on edge – I was on high alert and couldn't switch off when I tried. No amount of sleep seemed to fix it, and my hyper-alertness meant that sleep became harder the more exhausted I became.

It seems I am not alone in my zombie state. It looks like I could muster enough recruits to form a zombie army of burned-out brains. The actor Sandra Bullock described a similar loss of brain functioning: 'I'm so burned out, I'm so tired and I'm not capable of making healthy, smart decisions, and I know it.' It also looks like Beyoncé was fumbling along with her semi-functioning brain when she said: 'It was beginning to get fuzzy, I couldn't tell which day or which city I was at.' Welcome to the zombie army, Beyoncé.

Dimension 2: Increased mental distance from/ negativism or cynicism related to one's job

Well, anyone who knows me knows I am a (I believe healthy) cynic, but when I was burned out I lost all my enthusiasm, which normally counterbalanced my cynicism. I couldn't feel excited and engaged with what I was doing, nor what I was planning. I felt removed from things I'd previously been enthused by. I'm usually full of new ideas, but just thinking about doing anything new was exhausting and terrifying as I was struggling with my basic day-to-day tasks. My creativity diminished alongside my ability to function. I couldn't feel enthusiastic because I was just trying to get through the days – and enthusiasm requires energy, which I didn't have.

Now let's talk negativity. My brain could have talked to you all day about negativity. All brains have a negative bias (see the Baumeister, 2001, psychology paper 'Bad is stronger than

What is burnout?

good' if you want to read more about this).⁷ But boy, oh boy, when your brain goes into zombie mode, the negativity hosts a takeover and becomes a key driving force in your semi-functioning brain. It's well documented in scientific literature that when your brain is depleted, depressed or anxious, your natural tendency towards negativity increases, so it's no surprise this happens in burned-out brains too. My negativity ninja was kicking and screaming at me all day – at all the things I couldn't do or should have been doing. Seeing success on social media reflected all the things I wasn't doing or achieving. I knew I was a fantastic zombie, but clearly I was a terrible wife/mother/employee/author/daughter/worker (delete as appropriate, in fact just keep them all as the negativity was pervasive) because I wasn't functioning in the roles like I used to or wanted to.

I felt like life was out of control and I was failing at it, because in some ways I was – I was certainly failing myself. My negativity made me feel even more negative: I felt bad about being negative and dragging everyone else down around me (I wasn't, but this was how I perceived it).

Emma Gannon described something similar around her experiences in her Substack:

*This was the problem. I'm normally quite positive. I was in a shame spiral. I had swallowed that message from childhood whole: that if I wasn't positive, happy and productive then I wasn't of value.*⁸

Dimension 3: Reduced personal efficacy

Yes, for sure. I was ineffective at pretty much everything. Lots of people wouldn't have noticed this, because I was able to achieve at work to the standard I wanted to. The results looked good, but people couldn't see the extra effort I was putting in behind the scenes to achieve this or the detrimental impact of using all my energy to maintain my standards. Nor could they see what was lost as result of being a depleted battery, a zombie or that back-of-the-oven crispy chip in all other areas off my life. My cognition was slowed, my memory lapsed on an hourly basis, my communication was stilted and my attention was smashed to smithereens, taking with it my identity. I was ineffective at even basic tasks, including remembering to feed myself, drink water and take breaks (actually I was always rubbish at taking breaks – bit of a clue to one of the causes right there!). I was certainly ineffective at even more important tasks: parenting (sorry for all the beige meals, kids), friending, being fun or even being myself. Things that I would have enjoyed in the past became difficult. Nearly all aspects of me were blunted or crushed by the seeping exhaustion. I couldn't function like normal and in losing my abilities, I felt I had lost my identity and my worth. I didn't know who I was anymore, and this became a confusing fugue from which I couldn't escape.

Katherine May's description of her burnout from her Substack 'The Clearing' resonated with how I felt:

> *My brain was endlessly foggy, and I was spending my days harried, unsure what to focus on next. Whatever it was seemed urgent, but also beyond my reach. I wasn't sure what I was doing anymore.*[9]

What is burnout?

How do you know you are burned out?

Please note: It can be difficult to work out whether you are experiencing burnout or if other factors are contributing. A full assessment with a healthcare professional can help determine this, look at other possible reasons for how you feel and help you access appropriate support.

WHAT ARE YOUR SYMPTOMS?

Each of us has a different brain, different body, different experiences and different lives. This means that how burnout presents in you will most likely vary from the next person and be unique to you. In the depth of my burnout I asked on my Instagram about symptoms other people had experienced and themed them to create an illustration. These symptoms went beyond the traditional description of burnout, and this is also reflected in scientific papers that ask people about their experiences of burnout.[10]

I've adapted this to help you think about your burnout symptoms under the three dimensions of burnout. Use the illustration overleaf along with the exercise on pages 23-24 to think about which apply to you and add any additional symptoms you are experiencing. There is some debate about the nature and extent of symptoms you need to meet the burnout criteria.[11] The most commonly used burnout measure, the Maslach Burnout Inventory,[12] specifies you need to have symptoms across all three dimensions. I have added burnout measures to the notes on page 292 if you want to explore this further.[13]

BURNOUT

Emotional + Physical Exhaustion
- Tired all the time
- Brain shuts down
- Slow + lethargic

Detachment + Cynicism
- ↑ negativity
- Disengaged
- Hopeless

Reduced Efficacy
- Tasks take more time + effort
- Slower thinking
- Loss of purpose
- Feeling ineffective
- Self doubt

"I'm on fire!"

"Wish I could be that bright again!"

emotional impact
- Overwhelm
- Bigger emotional reactions
- Guilt + Shame
- Lack of enthusiasm
- Sense of failure
- Irritability

behaviour impact
- Loss of interest
- Withdrawal from people and activities
- Reduced enjoyment
- Loss of sense of humour

cognitive impact
- Difficulty with:
  - concentrating
  - decision making
  - switching off
  - planning
  - problem solving
  - motivation

physical impact
- Health problems
- Sleep issues

What is burnout?

Anti-burnout Exercise 1: Understanding your symptoms

List your current symptoms under the three categories of burnout, then add any additional symptoms on the next page.

1. Feelings of energy depletion or exhaustion:

   ....

   ....

   ....

   ....

2. Increased mental distance from/negativism or cynicism related to your job:

   ....

   ....

   ....

   ....

3. Reduced personal efficacy:

   ....

   ....

   ....

   ....

Physical symptoms:

....

....

....

Emotional symptoms (changes in how you feel):

....

....

....

Behavioural symptoms (changes in what you do):

....

....

....

Cognitive/thinking symptoms:

....

....

....

Other symptoms:

....

....

....

What is burnout?

IS YOUR 'WORK' CAUSING YOU STRESS?

According to the WHO diagnostic manual and research definitions, to be defined as burnout, the symptoms you experience should be related to your work/workplace:

Burn-out refers specifically to phenomena in the occupational context and should not be applied to describe experiences in other areas of life.[14]

Maslach tells us 'this is a workplace problem rather than a worker problem',[15] which means it's about the chronic stress that work causes an individual and the impact it has on them. Therefore, if someone is experiencing high rates of all the three dimensions – exhaustion, cynicism and inefficacy – because of WORK stress, that indicates they are burned out.

We've already looked at your burnout presentation, so now let's turn to whether it was a result of work. Okay, nice and easy: If your chronic stress or symptoms relate to work then you must be burned out. Hold on, though – what actually *is* work? The waters start to muddy when we dig in to how we conceptualize work.

First, let's think about the term 'work' or 'workplace'. They may bring to mind classic cubicles in an office, like the ones seen in *The Office* sitcom and films like *9 to 5* (and, an extreme example, in *Severance*) with a management structure in place. And I think that's what will come to mind for most people – an office-like environment of some description, or at least a building like a hospital, a restaurant, or school or clinic with some level of hierarchical structure or management. When I read articles or books about burnout, it seems, most often, this is what the author envisages and targets their advice at.

But is this really what work means in the 21st century? What workplaces are has shifted significantly in recent times, and they might now be your home, a café, even the online world. The systems and structures (if they do exist) might be remote, rather than a tangible person and structure, or you might be your own system if you are self-employed (which is on the rise). And what is work? Is it just the stuff we get paid for, or are we missing out important parts of our life that constitute work, such as study, education, caring or other unpaid labour, which can contribute to burnout too? To accurately understand burnout and the factors that contribute to it, I believe we need to widen our perception of work and the workplace.

How should we define 'work' in our modern world?

Studies looking at change in work in the 21st century argue that work can no longer be primarily defined in terms of place, employment, productivity or remuneration, and that our traditional view of it doesn't adequately capture its contemporary nature, or the diversity of the forms it takes.[16]

There has been a vast amount of research recently looking at unpaid labour, showing that it has traditionally been disregarded, which leads to society minimizing this type of work and the potential impact it can have. Research tells us that unpaid work (such as parenting, care work and domestic work) is often perceived as low value and is invisible in mainstream economics, and that this is underpinned by entrenched patriarchal institutions and national accounting systems that fail to factor in women's total contributions.[17] Of course, historically much of this work has, and continues to done, by

What is burnout?

women, which may go some length to explain why women are more at risk of burnout.[18] Reports have also concluded that disregarding this unpaid work can increase stress and contribute to burnout and poor mental health.[19] This means we really can't disregard it in a book about burnout – we need to value it, recognize it as work and see it as a potential contributor to burnout, because that's what the research says!

For the purposes of this book, we will consider work in a broad sense: as paid employment in all the various forms it takes in the modern world and as unpaid employment, including those forms of work that have often been disregarded, such as parenting, caring and domestic work. We will also include other things we intuitively know are work, such as studying, volunteering and things that feel like work to us, such as managing a chronic illness.

HOME LIFE MATTERS TOO

Whether we should really be focusing on work alone is also up for debate. How many of us can clearly separate our work and home life? Often the division between the two is blurred and it is the mixing of or tension between home and work life that creates stress. A 2024 study[20] challenged the belief that burnout is primarily work related. It found that factors in our personal life were also linked to burnout, concluding that we should also consider how individual-level and non-work factors contribute. This makes sense to me, because it was a combination of work (paid and unpaid) and multiple other factors that contributed to my burnout. The weight of everything together added to my stress levels.

So, when you consider what contributes to how you feel, I think we need to consider work in its broader, more modern sense as well as looking at the rest of your life. While some academics may disagree, from my clinical experience I firmly believe burnout can arise from attempts to meet obligations and demands across the spectrum of life. At its heart, it is a stress-related issue, and work factors, in the widest sense, along with meeting other obligations, often cause cumulative stress that contributes to how we are feeling.

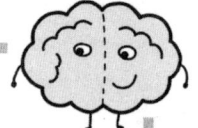

Brian the Brain reflections

- What does work look like to you?
- What paid work do you do?
- What unpaid work do you do?
- What else constitutes work to you?
- Has your work been causing stress recently (either due to the workload or other factors)?
- What other obligations do you have to meet that have contributed to cumulative stress?
- Is there tension between your home/work roles that creates stress?

Are you really burned out or is something else going on?

The honest answer for you is I don't know, and you may not yet either, but you do need to find out. The link between burnout and both physical and mental health conditions is complex and most likely bidirectional, and of course you can experience both physical and mental health concerns AND burnout at one time.

What is burnout?

In terms of physical health, it can be a complex picture.[21] While it is the case that burnout, and the inevitable chronic stress that is part and parcel of it, can contribute to the development of a range of health difficulties (more in Chapter 5), burnout can also make you more prone to illness and physical aches and pains. In addition, experiencing illness of any description is stressful, often time consuming and exhausting, and may add to your load, therefore contributing to the development of burnout. At the same time, fatigue is a common symptom of many health conditions and I have worked with people who discovered they have a physical health issue that explains how they feel, and therefore fatigue improved with treatment. For example, fatigue is a key symptom of conditions such as B12 or iron deficiency, or hypothyroidism, and often energy levels can return to normal if these are treated. As you can see, this is a complex picture that might need untangling.

If you are experiencing exhaustion, I would recommend getting checked out by a medical professional to answer the question of whether there is a physical health concern contributing to how you are feeling (and also to pick up any other conditions that may have resulted from the chronic stress). Burnout is often defined by excluding other potential causes, and for me this included a scree of blood tests and assessments that ruled out other physical health possibilities along with the inevitable question, 'Have you been stressed recently?' To which I answered, 'Er, yes, quite a bit I guess.'

Brian the Brain reflections

- What are your physical symptoms?
- What do you need to get checked out?

COULD IT BE A DIFFERENT MENTAL HEALTH ISSUE?

Please note: If you are feeling very hopeless or having suicidal thoughts, I would recommend immediately accessing a healthcare provider for assessment.

It's interesting that WHO doesn't categorize burnout as a mental disorder; they categorize it as relating to the environment. I believe this is to place the onus on the system that is causing stress, effectively removing blame from the individual or the burden on the individual to change. But to me, as a clinical psychologist, the picture is bit more complex. Let me explain.

The question I asked myself was this: Is this actually burnout I am experiencing or a mental health difficulty? I wondered if I was telling myself I was burned out because society viewed it as a more socially acceptable explanation for what I was feeling. We can't escape that, while mental health difficulties are unfairly stigmatized, suffering as a result of being busy is more likely to be seen as badge of honour in a society that values achievement and productivity. Look how hard I worked! Look how caring I was! Look how far I went to do a good job! Look how I suffered as a result of my efforts! Now don't get me wrong, I absolutely do not think these things about mental health difficulties, and I certainly didn't think my burnout was in any way glamorous or that it portrayed me in any special light. But I did doubt myself and wondered if I was just trying to define myself in a more socially acceptable way than face up to the perhaps more stigmatized label of mental illness.

Could a mental health condition explain how I was feeling? Maybe I was depressed or anxious. There are large overlaps between burnout and mental health conditions. Many of the symptoms overlap, and both burnout and other mental health conditions can result from chronic stress. Studies have shown that around 50 per cent of people who experience burnout also meet the criteria for depression. It's not clear whether this is cause or effect (it's likely both).[22] The impact of burnout can also lead to other mental health difficulties. I mean, being burned out can be depressing. The exhaustion sucks the joy out of nearly everything and it can feel like you are wading through a puddle of sinking sand you may never escape from. It can also be anxiety-provoking. Not being able to sleep, worrying about where your normal self has gone and whether you will be able to do what you have or want to do, or be the person you want to be.

I also know all too well from the many people I have worked with that experiencing a mental health condition can be stressful and demanding, using your resources and therefore contributing to burnout. In addition (just like burnout), many people I see with mental health difficulties experience them because of the stressful environment they are in, and things improve when their context changes. There are many ways that mental health conditions and burnout can cross over and sometimes it may only be possible to extrapolate what's going on with a full assessment by a health practitioner, such as a clinical psychologist.

Now I had a bit of an advantage here, as I know quite a lot about mental health, having worked in it for over twenty years, so I knew from looking at my own formulation (that's how a clinical psychologist understands someone's presentation) that the main trigger was chronic stress, characterized by an intensive period of work intertwined with my multiple other roles, wrapped up with the pandemic. In addition, I was able to see that my symptoms were highly consistent with burnout definitions. Yes, I could be anxious and sad because of how I felt, but these feelings were predominantly secondary to the exhaustion and other symptoms of burnout.

Building your own understanding might help you work this out for yourself but it's not always clear cut, so I would recommend that if you've been struggling with how you've been feeling and it's impacting on your day-to-day life, it's always best to see a doctor to assess this fully. In addition, therapy can be a helpful tool, and there's some evidence that medication may help with some of the symptoms, so it is worth exploring these options.

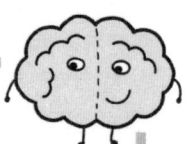

Brian the Brain reflections

- How would you describe your mental health currently on a scale of 0-10 (0 being very poor, 10 being very good)?
- How would you rate your mood on a scale of 0-10 (0 being very low mood, 10 being very good)?
- What about your anxiety levels (0 being anxious most of the time, 10 being very rarely anxious)?
- How is this impacting your day-to-day functioning?
- Do you need to take immediate action around how you are feeling OR do you need to get your mental health assessed further?
- How will you do this? For example, you could explore employee assistant programmes or speak to a health professional.

Building an understanding of where you are on the burnout scale

Whether you are burned out, becoming burned out or trying to protect yourself from burnout, it's important to understand what's going on. This includes any difficulties you are experiencing and any factors that are contributing to this feeling. In the next chapter, we are going to build your own personalized burnout formulation to help you assess where you are in terms of burnout.

For the time being, we are going to look at burnout on a scale - are you experiencing some symptoms and at risk of burnout or already in full-blown burnout? This can be used at any stage of the burnout spectrum, from burned-out crisp to noticing your flame dwindle, to proactively taking steps to keep your flame alive. At earlier stages of burnout you tend to have a few symptoms, or meet one or two of the dimensions. The later stages are when you meet all three dimensions and will have a greater amount or more pronounced symptoms. The scale is based on research into burnout stages[23] and will help you identify where you are now so you can:

- Protect yourself from burnout.
- Pick up on the early signs that you might be becoming burned out.
- Recognize if you are in full burnout.

We will expand this more into the full story of your burnout in Chapter 2, but for now let's think about your burnout scale. You can do something to be anti-burnout at every stage, including preventative action when you are not burned out.

The Anti-Burnout Book

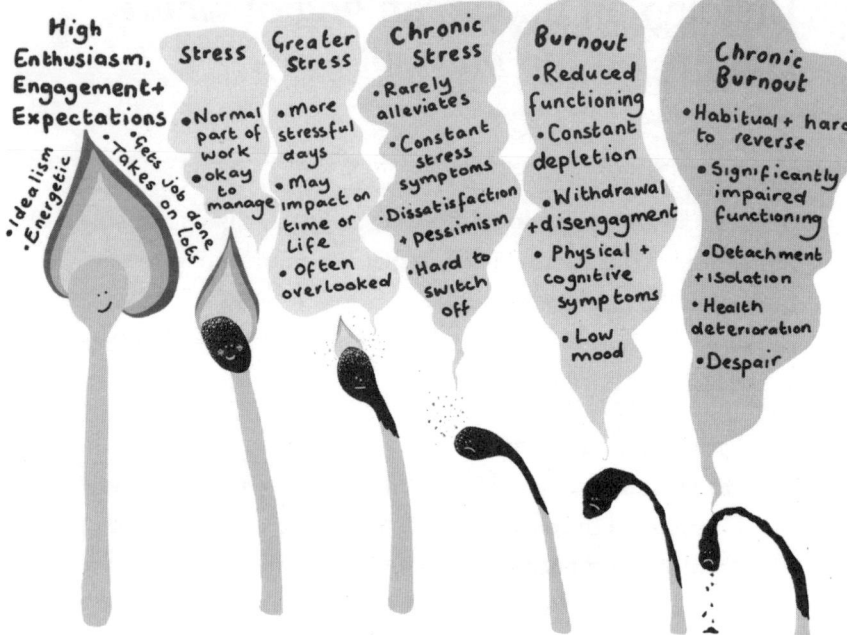

Anti-burnout Exercise 2:
Use the burnout scale above to identify which stage you are at

What are your signs you are at the different stages of the scale? You may not know this yet but fill in what you can. As you read through the book, think about what helps at different stages; for example, what keeps your flame alight and what helps when it starts to dwindle or is fully extinguished.

Anti-burnout takeaways

- Burnout is defined as experiencing work-related stress that has impacted on three areas: 1. Exhaustion; 2. Cynicism and negativity; 3. Reduced personal efficiency.
- When you think about work, you need to include paid and unpaid labour, and consider all other obligations and aspects of your life that contribute to your stress levels and load.
- Forming a clear picture of your symptoms can be a start to making sense of what's going on (see Exercise 1).
- There is a complex relationship between burnout and physical conditions, and it's important to have physical symptoms assessed by a medical doctor.
- There is also a complex relationship between burnout and mental health conditions and, if you are unsure if you are experiencing another mental health condition, it's important to have this assessed by a medical professional.
- If you are burned out, therapy or other treatments can be an important part of your recovery. Speaking to a healthcare professional can help clarify if you are burned out and help you access support.
- If you are feeling unable to participate in daily life at all, feel hopeless or are having suicidal thoughts, STOP reading now and seek help urgently.
- Understanding your burnout scale can help you understand which stage of your journey you are at. It can also help you spot the early signs and take preventative action.

Chapter 2
Building a burnout tree: Understanding what contributes to burnout

When you look up factors that cause burnout, you often see lists of negative workplace factors that create a toxic and stressful environment that is difficult to work in. Now, I have experienced plenty of toxic workplaces in the past, but it was not while I was working in one that I burned out. In fact, my manager was supportive and my colleagues were compassionate, engaging and had the same values as me. The work was energizing and meaningful and – at least in comparison to other roles I've had – I didn't think it was overly stressful (although, of course, working in healthcare through a pandemic was inherently so).

Above and beyond this, I was doing something exciting and thrilling that I could never have imagined would be part of my life: I was an author! I was writing books and being invited to take part in interesting book-related events. I didn't fit the profile of a downtrodden worker, crushed by their workplace and trudging through meaningless work that didn't engage them or value them (psychologically or monetarily). In fact, it was the opposite: I was too engaged. I felt lucky. There was so much interesting work coming my way that I was busy with meaningful tasks all the time. I used to say, if you looked at my life from the outside it would have seemed like the dream life – doing something I loved and being valued for it. At the same time, shame says: 'You are so lucky, look at your life – you should be grateful. There is no reason for you to feel bad or burn out.' Yet, I did.

What was the problem, then?

Ultimately, I was doing too much work, too much of the time, with too little time to rest. While each thing might not have felt hugely stressful in itself, the overall sheer number of things produced cumulative stress, with very little reprieve. I was wired, and my energy switch was ON most of the time, with very little time in OFF mode. In addition, my work life wasn't the end of my obligations. I am also a mother and wife and friend and daughter and sister and household planner and school email coordinator and emotional regulator of children and main family chef and shopper and bedtime book reader and family problem solver and holiday planner and health coordinator. Oh, I forgot the pandemic, so I was also home teacher (a rubbish one, if you ask my kids). I could go on, but I'm sure you've got the point!

For all of us, our obligations don't end when we leave the workplace. We don't have this mythical work–life balance where we leave the stressful workplace to a relaxing dreamscape of a life where we can switch off. In fact, for many of us – home workers, home schoolers, self-employed – work and home life are difficult to separate at all. Our 'must dos' continue in both landscapes, sometimes crossing over or merging, and our ongoing obligations across our whole life-scape can create stress. The cumulative demands can add to the pile of pending 'to dos' and weight on our shoulders, leading to burnout.

Am I to blame for my burnout?

As you've probably picked up from my shame narrator (let's call it Shane because it helps to externalize shame from myself), I experience a degree of shame around my burnout narrative. Not just because I'm a clinical psychologist or because I should have seen it coming (because it was so obvious when I look back). In fact, Shane visits most when I look at the causal factors of my burnout, because these weren't systemic factors out of my control, like working in a toxic environment or workplace bullying. They were, for the most part, things I chose to do. It was hard to feel sorry for me: nothing particularly bad had happened and many, many, many people had it far worse than me. I absolutely recognized how lucky I was (perhaps to the point where I sometimes minimized my own experiences). I was plainly the architect of my own burnout and there was nobody to blame but me. Yes, it WAS all my fault, and yes, that was Shane speaking. In reality, even though it *feels* like it was all my fault, there were lots of different risk factors at play.

Let's break this down a bit. If we put Shane aside, was it really all my fault? I clearly had behaviours, beliefs and coping styles that research tells us put us at risk of burnout. For example, I am bad at asking for help (ironic, I know, given that I help people for a living – but that's common in caring professionals). I'm definitely bad at taking breaks and prioritizing rest. Was my worth tied into productivity and achievement? Probably. Did I consider myself lazy if I was relaxing or not feeling busy and pressured? Definitely. My coping style is to persevere and keep going, tackling things until they are done, which has been helpful in the past but just wasn't in this situation, because there was no end to the tasks and I could never be 'done'.

There were also multiple other contextual risk factors going on in my life that contributed to my burnout, such as: my gender, systemic beliefs about domestic labour, high workload demands, to name a few. So of course it wasn't all about me. Yes, there were factors about me that were an important part of the mix, but the overall picture was much, much bigger than just me, and the same will apply to you.

ARE YOU TO BLAME FOR YOUR BURNOUT?

While I wouldn't have blamed anyone else for their story, like many people who experience burnout, self-blame and shame come along as an unwanted 'plus one'. I believe the definition of burnout (see Chapter 1) tries to reduce this blame by clearly locating the issue in the system in which we live and work. It's effectively saying, 'It's not your fault, it's the system that needs to change.'

Now that's easy to see and understand if you work in a system with clear, identifiable problems, such as a toxic workplace, bullying or harassment (but even then, I often see people blame themselves for what happened to them). However, it can be more difficult to see this if the system is wider than your immediate environment, or if it is not so obviously broken. In this case, the impact is more insidious. From my clinical experience, in this scenario we are even more likely to blame and shame ourselves. However, we need to recognize that the systems and context around us always play a role in the development of burnout.

So, the answer is of course you are not to blame for your burnout; it happened because of a complex mix of person, place, context and time. Yes, there will be personal aspects that contributed (your traits, behaviours and beliefs), but YOU are only one part of the story. It is the mix of these personal factors and context that is critical. In fact, your personal factors may have only become problematic because of the specific situation you were in. It's critically important to recognize your personal factors that played a part, but it is NEVER just down to you. It's NOT your fault and it is factually incorrect to blame yourself. It's also unhelpful and can block you from moving forward.

REMOVING YOURSELF FROM THE 'SHANE' SPIRAL

Ultimately, blame and shame are not helpful, as they inherently make us hide and shrink away from understanding and sharing our experiences. Ironically, this makes shame grow. To shift away from blame, it is more helpful to think about recognition and responsibility:

- Recognition of the internal and external factors that contribute to burnout.
- Responsibility to understand what contributes to how we are feeling and shift the factors that we have the power to, so that burnout is less likely to get its fiery claws into us and make us shrivel to a crisp of a person.

Being anti-burnout is about recognizing what contributes to your burnout (or risk of burnout) and holding yourself responsible to take action to protect yourself from future burnout.

Building a burnout tree

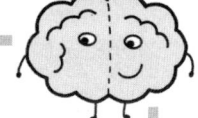

Brian the Brain reflections

- Are you blaming yourself for what has happened?
- How does this blame show up?
- Do you feel shame about your burnout story?
- What does your shame say to you?
- What aspects of your story do you feel shameful about?
- How does shame impact on what you do?
- Do you hide or mask aspects of yourself or your story because of shame? How does this affect you?

The burnout tree

Burnout is due to a complex interplay of personal and contextual factors. While they all contribute, it is the right (or I should say wrong!) mix of these factors that makes us burn out. I envisage all these factors as a tree. Let me explain.

Psychologists develop formulations to understand people's stories and difficulties and to guide which steps to take to help them. The tree is your burnout formulation, or story. It helps identify your **risk factors**, your **protective factors** and your **perpetuating factors** (what is keeping the issue going). It recognizes the **individual factors**, **context factors** and **wider systemic factors** that contribute to burnout. These factors are all intrinsically linked, and it is only by recognizing the whole picture that we can gain a full sense of your burnout picture and think about how we can make the tree flourish again.

Here's a breakdown of how this burnout formulation works:

- **The tree:** You are the tree, and each tree has core features such as age, role, gender, chronic ill health etc., some of which may put you more at risk. Your tree has to hold the weight of the stress created by the immediate environment and the wider system. Certain factors (including symptoms of burnout) might mean your tree is weakened at the moment and unable to deal with its normal levels of life stressors.
- **The ground:** The tree is rooted in the ground. The ground in which your tree grows represents the background factors which contribute to how it has grown so far, some of which may place you at greater risk of burnout.
- **The roots:** These are what keep you grounded. They are your protective factors against burnout or that help you get better. These can be your beliefs, your behaviours, your helpful coping strategies and the helpful parts of your context, such as supportive friends. We want to increase these to help protect you or move you out of burnout.
- **The branches:** These are your personal factors that contribute to your risk of or perpetuate burnout: how you cope, your beliefs, how you behave. Your branches interact with the things sitting on them. We want to target these to reduce your risk or help you recover from burnout.
- **The things sitting in your branches:** These are the stressors that contribute to burnout, creating demand and weight in your life. If you don't have the strength to hold them up, they can weigh your tree down, weaken it and cause structural stress and damage. Short term, your tree can recover quickly. But if stressed over a longer period of time, it can take longer to heal and be more difficult, but not impossible, to generate regrowth.

The Wider Environment

The Weather
your context

Stressors
The weight in your tree

your branches

ANTI-BURN OUT

your tree

your roots

the ground

- **The environment:** Finally, your tree exists in an environment which changes over time. This also influences how the tree grows, how much it can take root and what lands on it. Supportive environments nurture your tree and reduce the weight on its branches. Unhelpful environments tend to create more stress. We can think of the environment on two levels: the weather and the wider environment.
    - **The weather:** This is your immediate context, the situations that surround you day-to-day. Your work, your home, your family, your town, your culture, your religion. These factors can create stress and add more weight to your branches, or they can strengthen your tree and help support the weight it is holding.
    - **The wider environment:** These are systemic factors, which can include the wider political, societal and cultural context. They usually seem less tangible and out of our control, so we may dismiss their influence or feel helpless about how to tackle them. However, they also intrinsically influence how our trees grow; they create our social norms and influence what we believe and how we behave. They can also reduce or create stress. It's therefore important to consider how these wider factors influence our picture, or tree.

All of these factors are intrinsically linked, and only by recognizing the full picture can we gain a proper sense of your burnout story and think about how we can make your tree flourish again.

YOUR STORY

Now, your tree may be burned and shrivelled, or it may just be starting to weaken under the weight of the things in its branches, but wherever you are in your burnout journey it's important to understand the factors contributing to where you are and why you got there, because understanding your story gives you power.

Humans understand our lives through stories, and having a cohesive story joins all these confusing bits of information in our brain in a clear, structured way, which is comforting, less stressful and easier to understand and communicate. Secondly, it gives you the power to know what to do to help yourself. If we understand the contributing factors, we can work out how and where to focus our minimal energy to protect or relight our fires. We can identify where to start, what are the quick wins, what is within our control to target and which actions will have the greatest impact.

As you've probably guessed from my story, burnout doesn't announce itself with a great, explosive pyrotechnic bang. It's normally a slow, insidious burn, gradually fading you away until you reach a critical point. It's hard to notice and intervene early, but understanding our story gives us the power of awareness, so we notice when our tree starts to weaken and when action is needed. This knowledge is important for protecting ourselves now and in the future.

Now, let's start building your tree so you can take this power into your own hands to help it flourish and become more resistant to burnout.

The Great Big Blazing Burnout Quiz

Welcome to the quiz where we will find out what has contributed to your burnout story and work out your 'burnout score'. We will go through a list of factors that have been shown to contribute to burnout.[1] I have listed these into rounds based on the categories in the tree picture, with a tick box next to each factor. This is a 'pick and mix' exercise – in each round, **tick the factors that are relevant to you, then score each round**. At the end, combine the scores to get your final burnout score. Afterwards we'll add the factors you identify to your burnout tree, so we start to build your personal burnout story.

You won't identify with all these items, and that's okay because it's about identifying your unique mix of factors. You might have something in mind that you don't find on the list – that doesn't mean you are wrong, it's just that research tends to work with groups of people and it can't capture all individual experiences. So, if you have noticed a factor that has contributed to your burnout tree but is not on the list, add it anyway, because you are the expert in your own life and know more about your life than anybody else in this whole world.

A quick note: This is not a scientific questionnaire or validated measure.* It's just a fun, interactive quiz designed to really get you thinking about the relevant

---

* Most of these are based on scientific research, however I have also added some that I have commonly observed from my clinical experience of working with people with burnout.

Building a burnout tree

factors for your burnout tree and where you might need to target to become anti-burnout.

Round 1: Your tree (core features)

There are aspects of you that might make you more likely to experience burnout. These include life stages, roles and personal variables that make you more vulnerable. You can't always change these, but it's important to be aware of and recognize them, and to look at how they interplay with our stressors and protective and personal risk factors, to see if we can manage their impact differently.

- ❏ **Type of job:** Typically, high-demand or high-stress jobs are related to burnout, such as jobs where the mental effort through the day is high and has to be sustained, and when the demands are often impossible to complete in the hours available. The most common jobs cited in the research are healthcare workers (doctors, nurses, paramedics), social workers and teachers. However, many other roles could fit this profile, so tick if you think your role is a high-demand or high-stress job.
- ❏ **Life stage:** Certain stages of life may increase the risk of burnout. It's no surprise that parenting is one of them! Having a carer role (whoever you are caring for) is associated with high stress. There is also some evidence that burnout is more likely to occur during perimenopause or menopause. Give yourself a tick if you're a parent, an extra tick if you have young children, another if you're caring for older relatives or other people, and another tick for perimenopause or menopause, for good measure!

- ❑ **Career stage:** Being earlier in your career, whatever your line of work, may make you more at risk of burnout, probably because of a combination of self-doubt, along with doing everything for the first time. Female workers later in their career (over the age of 55) may also be at higher risk.[2]
- ❑ **Gender:** There is some evidence that females are more likely to burn out.[3] This may be because of a higher likelihood of caring duties, higher mental and domestic loads, and a clash of work and family life. Tick if you identify as female.
- ❑ **Neurodiversity:** There is evidence that people with a range of different neurodiverse labels may be at greater risk of burnout.[4] We'll explore this in more detail in Chapter 8. This may be because of cognitive or behavioural factors related to the diagnosis that increase mental effort, but it may also be about the environment you are in, which does not accommodate or meet the needs of neurodiverse individuals.
- ❑ **Health:** Experiencing illness (mental or physical) or chronic pain can create stress and reduce your capacity.

Now score round 1. Tot up your total number of ticks for round 1 here _____ and add that number into the score box on page 55.

Round 2: The ground (background factors)

These are things that have happened in your past which may make you more at risk of burnout. Our past influences the present through our physiology, belief systems, our thinking and cognitive styles, how we cope and how we behave in

Building a burnout tree

different contexts. We are not going to go into each of these in detail, but I have added resources at the back of this book if you wish to read more. In addition, if you are concerned about how these factors are impacting on you and your presentation, then I would recommend seeking support from a psychological or healthcare professional.

- **Difficult childhood:** Childhood is the time when our beliefs about ourselves, other people and the world develop. Having a stressful and difficult childhood (often called Adverse Childhood Events, or ACEs) can make us vulnerable to a range of health difficulties, including burnout.
- **Previous trauma:** Trauma is associated with emotional, cognitive and physical symptoms that might make you more vulnerable to burnout. These can include emotional vigilance, strong emotional reactions or suppression of emotional reactions, hyperarousal and a range of physical symptoms, such as exhaustion or sleep difficulties.
- **Previous negative experiences at work:** These may make us more wary and emotionally vigilant, which uses up our precious energy. We may feel we need to mask how we are feeling or have difficulty asking for support. We may have difficulty trusting co-workers or our employers, and we may not feel valued.
- **Chronic sleep difficulties:** If you have difficulty sleeping then you may not get the restorative rest you need, so your tree is fundamentally weakened and unable to hold as much in its branches.

Round 2 score: _____

Round 3: The branches (personal risk factors)

Tick any traits below that you think are relevant to you:

Personal characteristics:
- ❏ Perfectionism[5]
- ❏ Very self-critical/low self-compassion
- ❏ Tendency to internalize or blame yourself when things go wrong
- ❏ Low confidence in abilities (high level of imposter syndrome)
- ❏ Identity strongly tied into work
- ❏ High empathy or altruism

Beliefs:
- ❏ Beliefs around rest and self-care, e.g. viewing looking after yourself as self-indulgent or rest as a luxury
- ❏ Negative beliefs about yourself
- ❏ Beliefs about success based on achievements/status
- ❏ Feeling helpless to change your situation
- ❏ Shame around experiencing difficulties and failure

Coping styles:
- ❏ Avoidance
- ❏ Perseverance (this can often be helpful, but research indicates that persevering when we are overloaded or entering/experiencing burnout can become detrimental)
- ❏ Using alcohol or drugs to cope with stress
- ❏ Unwillingness to seek help

Behaviours:
- ❏ Difficulty switching off from work (in your mind or due to technology use, always having access to emails etc.)

- ❏ Not taking breaks/down time
- ❏ Responding to emotions by not acknowledging them, or hiding or suppressing them
- ❏ Tendency to ruminate when things go wrong

Round 3 score: _____

Round 4: The roots (things that protect you)

Think about the personal and wider protective factors that support you or help you cope on a day-to-day basis. I won't list everything here, but these are some key factors that can make your roots strong and protect you from burnout, reduce the impact and help you recover.

- ❏ Good social support (within and outside of work)
- ❏ Security in daily life (financial, emotional, physical)
- ❏ Strong boundaries between work and personal life (but let's recognize that for many people this is really difficult, particularly if we shift how we think about work, as described in Chapter 1)
- ❏ High levels of self-compassion
- ❏ Work that aligns with your values, a supportive workplace and a manageable workload

Each tick in this section should <u>deduct</u> 3 from your burnout score. Please think of any other additional protective factor that applies to you and log **-3 points for each**.

Round 4 score (amount to be subtracted from your existing score): _____

Round 5: The weight in your branches (stressors)

What's going on in your life that's causing stress? There is only so much weight your tree can take – if it has too much demand, and not enough capacity to deal with it, this can weaken your tree. At certain points in life you may have reduced capacity to deal with difficulties, yet you may not notice and continue to pile the same weight onto your tree. And sometimes the weight gets added in small doses incrementally, so you don't notice when you start to reach the tipping point. Each individual thing may not cause much stress in itself, but the combined weight weakens your tree.

Think about adding all the specific things that are causing you stress or using up your capacity. We can think of them in these categories:

- **Small stressors** that may not cause significant stress in themselves, but together create significant stress.
- **Large stressors** that overwhelm you immediately.
- **Stressors that seem out of control** when things feel beyond your control, or you feel unable to do anything about the demands. Separating your stressors into ones you can or can't control will help (more in Chapter 3).
- **Internal stressors** might be your constantly critical voice that shouts at you and weighs you down, or the non-stop ruminating that comes into your mind at night and keeps you awake.
- **Background noise** includes things going on in your life that use your capacity and require your energy. They may not feel particularly stressful but form part of the overall weight.

Now score the number of stressors in your tree on a scale from 0 (stress free) to 10 (loads of stress crushing your tree).

Round 5 score: _____

Round 6: The environment around your tree

Part 1: The weather: your immediate context

While most of the research looks at factors in traditional workplaces that cause stress, we can think about factors in relation to work in the widest sense and in our personal life.

Characteristics of your role:

- ❏ Unmanageable work overload/long hours
- ❏ Job insecurity
- ❏ Ambiguity of roles or unclear roles
- ❏ High level of emotional labour – e.g. dealing with complex emotional situations and trauma
- ❏ Imbalance between effort and reward (you don't feel rewarded for your role)
- ❏ Unfairness – e.g. people treated or paid differently for the same role

Characteristics of the culture:

- ❏ Culture of self-sacrifice – where you don't take breaks or rest
- ❏ Psychologically unsafe environment – where you do not feel safe to raise concerns or issues (see Chapter 6)
- ❏ Stigmatization of seeking help or having mental health difficulties

- ❏ Toxic/blame culture (shared belief systems and attitudes that influence behaviour)
- ❏ Value conflicts – where your values are challenged by the context you are in and/or are not being met

Characteristics of the people around you:
- ❏ Lack of support structures
- ❏ High levels of conflict
- ❏ Unsupportive leaders/family members/peers (or characteristics of those in your close environment – do they increase stress or support you to manage stress?)
- ❏ Lack of respect or trust
- ❏ Discrimination, bullying or harassment

Other characteristics of the work/life context:
- ❏ Struggling financially
- ❏ Environment not suited to your individual needs – e.g. for neurodiversity or disability
- ❏ Work and non-work conflict/interference – where your job interferes with your home life or vice versa
- ❏ Unsafe/uncomfortable physical environment (office/home etc.)

Round 6 Part 1 score: _____

Part 2: The wider environment

Below is a list of wider systemic factors that can contribute to overall stress and burnout. Have a think and tick those that you feel apply to you.

- ❏ Unsupportive and unsafe wider cultures – e.g. volatile political systems or risk to you due to political situation

Building a burnout tree

- ❏ Beliefs and attitudes towards illness, race, sex, disability etc.
- ❏ World events that create stress directly or vicariously – conflict, traumatic events, environmental issues
- ❏ Physical environment – e.g. secure housing, access to green space, air quality
- ❏ Social structures – e.g. lack of access to healthcare, education, childcare

Round 6 Part 2 score: _____

Congratulations! You have completed the Great Big Burnout Quiz. Now tally up your scores (**remember to minus the scores in Round 4 from your total**) and add it to this box:

Round	1	2	3	4 (minus)	5	6 (Pt.1)	6 (Pt.2)
Score							
TOTAL SCORE:							

Higher scores indicate you are more likely to be burned out or have a greater risk of burnout. Use the 'yikes scale' below for a general indication of how you are faring.

- **0 (or less)–19:** No yikes yet. Your tree seems to be holding up okay, with a manageable number of risk factors and stress. But you still need to keep an eye on these and manage them proactively to keep yourself in the 'no yikes' zone.

- **20-34:** Yikes, your tree has some risk factors and stress to hold up. Ensure you manage them so they don't weigh your tree down too much long term.
- **35-49:** Double yikes! There's a lot for your tree to hold right now. Is it managing or is it being crushed by the weight? Take action to manage this situation now!
- **50+:** Exponential yikes!! Has your tree toppled over? You've identified lots of factors that contribute to burnout – are you already in full zombie mode? Whether your tree is still bearing the weight or is totally crushed, action is needed.

While this exercise is just to help you think, and not a scientific questionnaire,* if you are scoring very highly and/or feel you are having difficulty functioning right now, this could be an indication that you may benefit from seeking help from a medical professional or other sources to support you.

Now you've done this, you can start building your burnout tree in the next exercise to help you better understand your story.

---

* A validated measure of burnout is included in the reading list at the back of this book if you do want to explore more.

Building a burnout tree

Anti-burnout Exercise 3: Build your burnout tree

Start to fill in your burnout tree. You can do this by sketching out your own tree based on the drawing on page 43 and/or by listing the factors on the following pages. This is an idea of what is contributing to your burnout. It can help you make sense of your story while directing you to where you can take action. If you have sought support from a psychologist, counsellor or therapist, then often they will build a formulation with you (although it probably won't look like a tree!).

It's okay if your tree is incomplete or you can't make sense of your picture initially. You can continue to build on it as you read this book. It can also be helpful to go through this with someone you trust, whether a colleague, family member or friend. Two brains can often help build a more comprehensive picture than one.

If you can't make any sense of your story at all, don't worry. We will speak about some of the specific factors you can start to tackle as we go. If you are finding this difficult, it may also be time to think about whether you need professional input to help you understand your burnout picture and what you need to happen to recover.

- **The tree (your core features such as age, role, gender, chronic ill health etc.):**

....

....

- **The ground (background factors):**

  ....

  ....

  ....

- **The roots (protective factors):**

  ....

  ....

  ....

- **The branches (personal risk factors):**

  ....

  ....

  ....

  ....

Building a burnout tree

- **The things sitting in your branches (stressors):**

  ....

  ....

  ....

  ....

- **The weather (immediate context):**

  ....

  ....

  ....

  ....

- **The wider environment (systemic factors):**

  ....

  ....

  ....

  ....

Anti-burnout takeaways

- Many people feel shame or blame themselves when they experience burnout. Shame thrives in darkness when we hide how we are feeling.
- Burnout is not your fault – you may have personal factors that contribute but they are part of a much bigger mix of factors.
- Recognizing that there are personal factors that contribute to burnout and taking responsibility to change them, when you can, is part of understanding burnout.
- It is important to recognize the bigger picture and the range of factors that put you at risk or have contributed to your burnout.
- Understanding all the different factors can help you make sense of your story and inform what you can do to help.
- The burnout tree is an exercise I have developed through my clinical practice to help understand the factors that contribute to someone who is at risk of or is experiencing burnout.
- Understanding your burnout tree can help you make sense of your story, know where to target your energy to recover and prevent future burnout.

PART 2
How to Avoid Burnout

Chapter 3

Under pressure: Stress, stress and more stress

Let me introduce you to my little friend who I got to know very well through burnout: Twitch. Or, to give her full posh name, Ocular Myokymia, which is a right-eyelid muscle contraction. Twitch came with me everywhere I went and grew bigger when I was stressed, tired or had lots on. She was usually just my little pet but sometimes became so strong she was visible to others. She even appeared on TV, when I went on the BBC to talk about my new book. Twitch was just one of the physical manifestations of my stress, because stress is not something imaginary – it's a real physical thing happening in your body and brain.

For example, when I was approaching burnout, the accumulation of stress was having multiple effects on my body beyond Twitch. Having been very healthy throughout my life, I started rapidly collecting symptoms, which then turned into conditions, which then turned into regular appointments, treatments, failed treatments and uncertainty. And I started going bald. Yes, you read that right – my hair started to fall out and I had an obvious bald patch that only an extreme side-parting could hide (unfortunate, as middle partings were trendy at the time; I looked highly uncool).

I also noticed that my attention and memory started to falter, and that planning and organizing seemed more difficult. This meant that other areas of my life that required time and effortful brain work lapsed. Life started to feel overwhelming, out of control and shameful (I'm telling you, Shane had a never-ending brain party), creating even more stress. I would say the impact of stress was stressful in itself.

We need to be serious about stress, because it can have serious implications for our health and life.

What do we mean by stress?

Stress is a good thing. Okay, hear me out here, because obviously it wasn't a good thing for me. But stress is an ubiquitous experience that we all have at different levels throughout life. It's just part of life, we can't avoid it. In fact, it's so ubiquitous that the brain is designed specifically to predict, respond to and adapt to stressors, which keeps us safe and healthy. This bodily response (which can sometimes feel really unpleasant) gets us through life. It directs our energy to where it is needed and helps us spot problems, recognize demands and achieve our goals. And if we keep stress at a manageable level (and allow ourselves to recover from it), it can even be helpful: we can feel energized and boosted; it can motivate and engage us; our body recovers (and sometimes even improves because it boosts our immunity) and gets back into a state of equilibrium afterwards. But sometimes, as in my case, there is too much stress, and we don't or can't always manage this. Let's delve further.

DEFINING STRESS

Well, I thought this would be the easy section of the book, but how wrong I was. Let's start from the beginning. In the 1930s, Hans Selye, an endocrinologist in Austria, came up with the term 'stress' to describe a physiological and emotional adaptive response.[1] The word 'stress' was derived from a Latin term meaning 'to draw tight' (which makes sense if I think about Twitch and how my neck muscles felt during burnout). Nowadays stress is spoken about so much that I feel it's one of those things we all kind of know about, but when we delve into it, it becomes a much more confusing picture. The language around stress is inherently confusing. When we refer to stress, we can mean lots of different things, such as events that make us stressed, the body's physical stress response or how we feel emotionally. There's lots of different terminology around stress that adds to the confusion: pressure, overwhelm, eustress (positive stress) tension, arousal. It's not surprising that the concept is confusing. It turns out, stress can be many different things to many different people; but that doesn't help us much. So, let's simplify it here for the sake of this book.

I'm not going to go into all the different theories and models – that's for a university lecture (but if you want to read about this, see the reference[2]). But I am going to break it down in the way I explain it to people I work with, so that we have a shared understanding.

In its simplest terms, stress is about pressure being exerted on something. Pressure puts things under strain. We experience stress (the feeling of tension or strain) because of the demands of life (stressors) and the resulting pressure they create. What we feel is due to our body's responses to these stressors (our stress response). Of course, there's a lot more complexity to it than this, because whether we experience stress and how we manage demands depends on a number of things, including our capacity and our beliefs and thoughts about that stressor. I like to think of stress as the name we use to describe how we feel, which is our experience of the bodily response to demands and pressure. So, let's break this down into its component parts.

Stressors

These are the demands of life that can cause stress (the weight on our branches). There can be lots of little things that by themselves are not stressful (micro stressors) that can add up to create a lot of pressure. Or sometimes one big stressor gets thrown at us that creates a lot of pressure (for example, a loved one being ill). Not all stressors are equal: some create more pressure – for example, those that feel out of our control and we feel helpless to change.

It's not just about having too much on; it's also about what we are missing. While it's obvious that a lack of money can create stress, having too little of other things can be a stressor too. We might lack the structure, interest, meaning or connection that humans need to thrive (the science shows that loneliness creates lots of stress[3]).

Stressors aren't just the current demands, either. We have an amazing power as humans to imagine the future and think about the past. Perhaps it's regret over decisions or memories of unhappy or traumatic events, or thinking about a future event that is going to happen – or even imagining events that may never happen! Even how you speak to yourself can be a stressor. Knowing your stressors is an important part of managing your stress.

Stress body response

To deal with demands, the brain and body need to prepare us for action. The brain needs to direct our energy and attention to the demands to deal with them, whatever they may be. This is our stress response, and it's going on all the time in our body and brain to keep us healthy and enable us to respond to and manage the world around us. But sometimes we may have a bigger response, if the stressor is bigger or if there are lots of things going on at once which means we feel more stressed. Ironically, I feel a bit stressed writing this section on stress – I'm feeling my shoulders tighten and my brain feels a bit jumbled, but it's currently at a level that feels manageable. The level of stress we are experiencing is really important, so let's look a bit more at that.

Levels of stress

The term 'stress' is often used to describe when stress becomes too much, when demands outweigh capacity (this definition is often used in scientific papers), or, in layman's terms, when you feel totally overwhelmed. However, we can feel different levels of stress: sometimes it can feel manageable; sometimes it can feel overwhelming. When it creeps up and reaches a high level, it can bubble over, overflow our capacity and become overwhelming, which can impact us in a number of unhelpful ways. It's important to recognize where your stress levels are to help you manage them. I find it helpful to use a 'demand and capacity' model of stress in my clinical work, to help understand levels of stress, what's contributing to them and how to manage them. Let's look at that now.

Under pressure

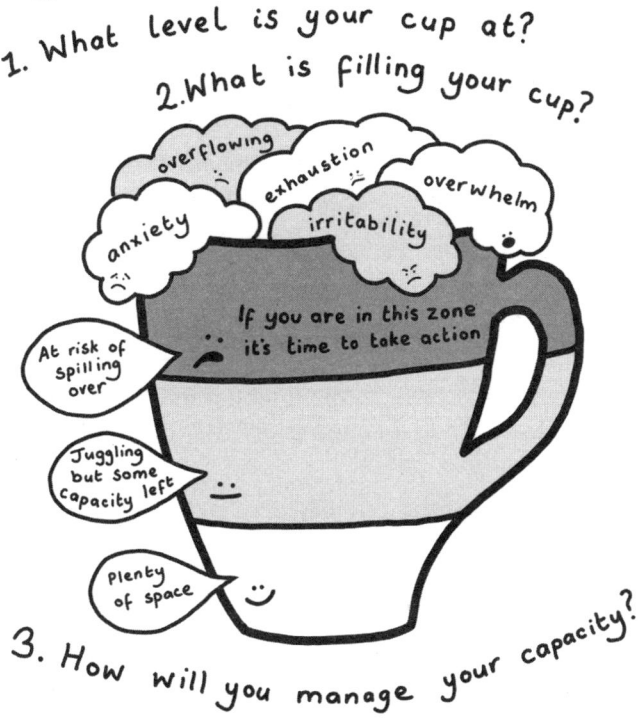

Anti-burnout Exercise 4: The capacity cup: managing your stress levels

This is a way of looking at stress using a 'demands and capacity' model that I first devised for a brain injury group I was running. It's based on the idea that we all have limited capacity, and that capacity fills up from the demands of life. As our capacity gets fuller, our stress levels rise. If the demands are greater than our capacity can hold, then our cup bubbles over: there is too much stress and we are in a state of overwhelm. We can use this regularly to notice our stress levels and then think about what we can do to both manage the stressors and find ways to increase our capacity (help us cope with them).

Step 1: Where is your capacity cup currently?
- Bottom layer: Feeling okay, calm
- Middle layer: Some stress but manageable
- Top layer: High levels of stress
- Bubbling over: Overwhelmed with stress

Steps 2-4 can be helpful at any time but particularly if you need to take action to manage stress.

Step 2: What are the stressors?

Write down all the demands currently filling your cup. Remember, these can be external or internal. If you are worrying about something constantly, that is a stressor too. Think about the following:

- Are there lots of little things going on (that may together create too much demand)?
- Are there big things causing a lot of stress?
- Is there too much of something (such as too much work that you can't do in the time available)?
- Are there things that are causing you worry?
- Is there something you feel you are lacking in your life (such as connection, interest, creativity)?

It can also be helpful to divide the stressors you identify into categories:

1. Causing you most stress.

2. Out of your control, which you feel helpless to do anything about.
3. Can be tackled easily – you might be able to take quick action here that makes you feel more in control.

Step 3: What steps can you take to manage these stressors?

Are you able to:

- Stop or reduce them?
- Problem-solve next steps?
- Talk them through with someone?
- Put a plan in place for how to deal with them?
- Cut back some of them?
- Ask other people to help?
- Find ways to manage the things you are worried about?
- Think of ways you can get support from other people?

Step 4: Are there other ways you can increase your capacity to help you cope better?

For example, you could take some time out, access your support network, eat healthily, take a walk or get a better night's sleep. These make you feel better overall and therefore help increase your capacity.

Step 5: Are there ways that you are coping that reduce your capacity?

Your coping mechanisms may increase your stress longer term (we'll look at this more in the Stress Fertilizer exercise on page 79).

When stress becomes unhelpful

Remember that body stress response I said was helpful? Well, it is, unless it keeps on going for too long and we don't let ourselves recover from it. Then, I hate to say, it becomes our worst enemy. It is the long-term firing of this response, with no time for our body and brain to recover, that leads to burnout.[4] And it doesn't stop there, as long-term chronic stress is linked to just about any illness in any body system you can think of, from the brain (increased mental health difficulties) to the veins (increased risk of hypertension and stroke) to the heart (increased risk of heart attack).[5] Once you start reading the list of conditions that the research tells us stress can lead to, it starts to, ironically, become stressful. You don't need a list of them here (but can find one in the references[6]) but it's enough to say that long-term, chronic, unmanaged stress is a really, really bad thing for you and your body. To reframe this (hey, that's what psychologists do!): it's very, very, very important to notice, understand and manage stress so it doesn't become chronic and cause all the problems, like, oh you know, perhaps burnout (and heeeeeeeere's my shame voice, Shane, again: 'What right do you have to tell people to manage their stress – you didn't exactly manage it, did you?').

THE HELPFUL BODY STRESS RESPONSE

Let's look a bit more at the body's response to stress and why it happens. I'm not going into micro-neuroscientific detail here (believe me, it's fascinating, but it could take up a whole book, so see Further Reading on page 306 if you want to read more[7]). Let's start with your brain: the amazing organ through which you experience and make sense of the world. It has many functions, but the overall point of your brain is thought to be

Under pressure

homeostasis,[8] which is basically keeping your body resources in check so that you stay healthy. To do this efficiently, it needs to look to the future. At its heart (or I should say *corpus callosum*, because that's kind of the centre of your brain), your brain is a predictive organ, constantly working out what is about to occur, to ensure you have the energy and resources you need to deal with whatever is coming your way. It is not the most mindful organ; it definitely DOES NOT live in the moment.

When your brain predicts you need more energy to deal with something, it fires up brain and body systems to get you ready for action. These systems are not uniquely about stress; they are firing all the time throughout your day and your life to deliver energy when you need it – to get you up in the morning, to deal with deadlines or to get you through that boring meeting. They are not responsible for stress, but they are an important part of it. The whole system description I will leave for neurology and physiology books (see page 306), but here's a brief overview of how your brain revs up your body for action.

When your brain predicts something is about to happen that you need energy to deal with (it makes these predictions based on memory and past experience), it sets off a chain of clever events:

> Your brain detector, or amygdala, has spotted that your brain has predicted you need to get ready for action, and sends signals to your hypothalamus, which communicates to your body via the autonomic nervous system (which has two parts: sympathetic and parasympathetic).

Your sympathetic nervous system is fired up and multiple hormones are released, including adrenaline, which surges through your body to energize you and get you ready.

This sets off a chain of events that fires up body systems that help you take action.

This process sets off a chain of multiple body responses, including:

– Your brain becomes more focused and threat-alert.

– Your pupils dilate to enhance your vision.

– Your heart beats faster to pump more blood around your body.

– Your blood pressure rises.

– Your immune systems boosts so you can heal faster if you get hurt.

– Your breath becomes quicker and shallower to get more oxygen to your body.

– Your body releases glucose to supply more energy into your bloodstream.

If you need this response to continue, this is followed by a secondary process that releases a further set of hormones, including cortisol, to keep these processes going. This is, effectively, your brain keeping its foot on the accelerator.

> At the same time other body responses – high-energy demand systems that you just don't need at this time – are deprioritized (for example, digestion and complex brain systems) so you can use energy effectively where it is really needed.

We are not always aware of this reaction, but when we are, we might label it as anxiety, stress or a range of other emotions. The process is often described as the 'flight or fight' (and sometimes 'freeze') response, and it helps you deal with stressors. In the short term, these responses all help us access the energy and resources we need to get through stressors and deal with threat and the everyday demands of life. I hope you can appreciate how clever your brain and body systems are, because without this response, we would not even get through the day. I told you it was a good thing – it's called the sympathetic nervous system because it's (supposed to be) sympathetic to the needs of your body. But, like many good things, it has a downside if it happens too much, and to explain this I'll hand you over to Britney Spears.

CHRONIC STRESS: 'DON'T YOU KNOW THAT IT'S TOXIC?'

You better believe Britney, because chronic stress is toxic for you, your brain and your body. If your brain keeps your stress system ramped up too much, for too long, with not enough recovery, then all those helpful effects start to become unhelpful, burning out your body and brain. Burn out is not an analogy: by keeping your stress response on high you are using up your energy and body resources, and your brain becomes depleted and no longer so adaptive.

This is because your very clever and sympathetic stress response is designed to manage shortish-term stressors, then switch off and balance this response with periods of recovery. This is achieved through the other part of our autonomic nervous system: the parasympathetic nervous system, often called the 'rest and digest' system. It puts the brakes on your stress response and helps you recover from stressors, by conserving energy and calming your brain and body the heck down. This system operates to heal your body from the period of high energy use. It's like plugging in your electric car to recharge – there's only so much energy it can use before it becomes depleted and needs to be topped up to continue functioning.

Now brace yourself, because this next bit is a scary read. Over-firing of brain systems means they become strengthened while other brain systems become depleted.[9] This can result in being on a constant state of high alert longer term and experiencing cognitive issues, such as poorer memory and reduced attentional capacity. Our brain predictions can also start to become faulty, so they no longer help us in the way they should, instead predicting threat and revving us up for it when there is none.[10]

Additionally, all the physical effects of stress impact health.[11] Long-term muscle tension can lead to musculoskeletal problems. The deprioritizing of body systems can lead to digestive issues and loss of libido. High blood pressure increases the chance of multiple diseases, including stroke and heart condition. Long-term cortisol impacts on multiple body systems, including your brain's memory systems. In an attempt to manage and provide energy, your body stores more fat and craves high carbs. Over-firing of the immune system can mean your very own clever protective system turns against you and targets your own body, which in turn is linked to multiple chronic illnesses, including auto-immune conditions and mental health issues. Even scarier is that this is just a snapshot, as long-term stress impacts multiple body systems resulting in various (ironically very stressful) symptoms, including my pet twitch and my hair loss (long-term stress can push hair growth into resting phase or the immune system can attack the hair follicles). The list goes on and on and on, and this means Shane the shame monster has a whale of time telling me about all the problems I have caused by not managing my stress well. Ultimately, long-term stress leads to multiple physical and mental health issues (all of which are underpinned by physical mechanisms). One of which, of course, is burnout.

> **Anti-burnout Exercise 5:**
> **Spotting the signs of toxic stress**
>
> Understanding your signs of stress can help you take early action. Think about how stress responses show up for you:
>
> 1. What are your signs of stress?
>
> Body signs: ....
>
> Thinking signs: ....
>
> Behaviour signs: ....
>
> Let's work out if this is toxic stress. This is indicated by long-term experience of stress signs, little reprieve from them and worsening of symptoms.

> 2. How long have these signs been going on for?
>
> 3. Are these signs always present or occur more often than not?
>
> 4. Have these signs been worsening (an indication of chronic stress) or become longer-term patterns of behaviour (e.g. social withdrawal or prolonged sleep difficulties)?
>
> 5. Are there other symptoms or signs you have been experiencing that may indicate chronic stress (e.g. shifts in mood, changes in cognition, health issues*)?

THE EXPONENTIAL GROWTH OF THE STRESS WEED

I like to view stress as a pervasive weed, as it has a nasty little way of creeping into our life without us noticing. It seems to grow exponentially compared to other plants, and sends off tendrils and shoots that keep it alive and create more weeds. It can also become all-pervasive, smothering the nice plants. It does this in a number of ways.

Firstly, the impact of stress and the very symptoms it creates can in themselves be stressful and create more stress. My hair loss was stressful and the number of symptoms I was experiencing created uncertainty and extra demands, using time and resources I did not have. My crappy memory, too,

---

* Remember! Please get any health issues or cognitive changes checked out by a medical professional who can help you understand whether stress is the cause.

was a constant source of stress – what had I forgotten? And my extra snappiness, irritability and short fuse (all classic signs of stress – sorry, kids) was not like me, and I felt guilty about this, which increased my stress.

Secondly, stress can feel overwhelming and lead us to neglect other areas of our life, which then become overwhelming in themselves and create more stress. We may not take time to look after our basic needs, which creates more stress for our body, or we may neglect other areas, which build up and create stress. For me, it was keeping on top of household tasks, and these grew to be an additional stressor. I also didn't take time to see friends, which not only made me feel guilty but it also took away things that might have reduced my stress.

Thirdly, the very way that stress impacts our brain and emotions ironically keep the stress going. For example, high threat alert and vigilance can lead to sleep difficulties, more focus on the negative stuff and the exponential growth of crappy thoughts.

In these ways, stress becomes like one of those never-ending circus mirrors (perhaps a cracked one, though), where stress creates stress, which then creates more stress and so on, *ad infinitum*. But we also need to take some responsibility for the stress weed, because sometimes we can unintentionally fertilize it with how we try to manage it.

Are you fertilizing the stress weed?

How we cope with stress can either help or hinder our stress, and our likelihood of burnout. There's lots of research across multiple psychology fields that demonstrates how coping styles affect how we manage.[12] To summarize, being kind to yourself and actively dealing with stressors – such as problem solving, seeking social support and talking things though – helps us to cope better. Conversely, being nasty and critical and passively dealing with stressors – such as avoidance, withdrawal and hiding difficulties – makes things worse. This means that how we cope with stress can help, or it can create a horrible vicious cycle where it undermines our ability to cope. These 'coping strategies' have the opposite effect: they stop us shifting into the recovery phase, keep us stuck in the stress response and create more stress. We unintentionally fertilize stress rather than suppressing its growth.

For example, one of my key coping strategies is to face things head on and get them dealt with. This is an active coping style most scientific papers will tell you is helpful, and it has worked well to help me manage short periods of high stress in the past. But as the nature of stress became more pervasive, demands increased and my capacity decreased (because I was getting burned out), this became a hugely unhelpful coping strategy for me. Too much perseverance meant I kept going, trying to tackle an impossible load and not stopping. I didn't give up, I soldiered on. Until I couldn't anymore.

There were other ways I fertilized my stress. I was so exhausted that I avoided people, because I knew I wasn't myself. I opted out of many things: family film nights, seeing friends or even responding to texts suggesting meeting up. I didn't want to join in, as people would get a wasted-away zombie version of me that wasn't much fun. However, in avoiding my support network, I was reducing the protective factors that keep me grounded. Stress was creating that vicious cycle.

Now let's look at how you cope with stress and ways you may unintentionally fertilize your stress weed (remember, what was once a helpful coping strategy may now not be), and how you can create helpful cycles that suppress your weeds instead.

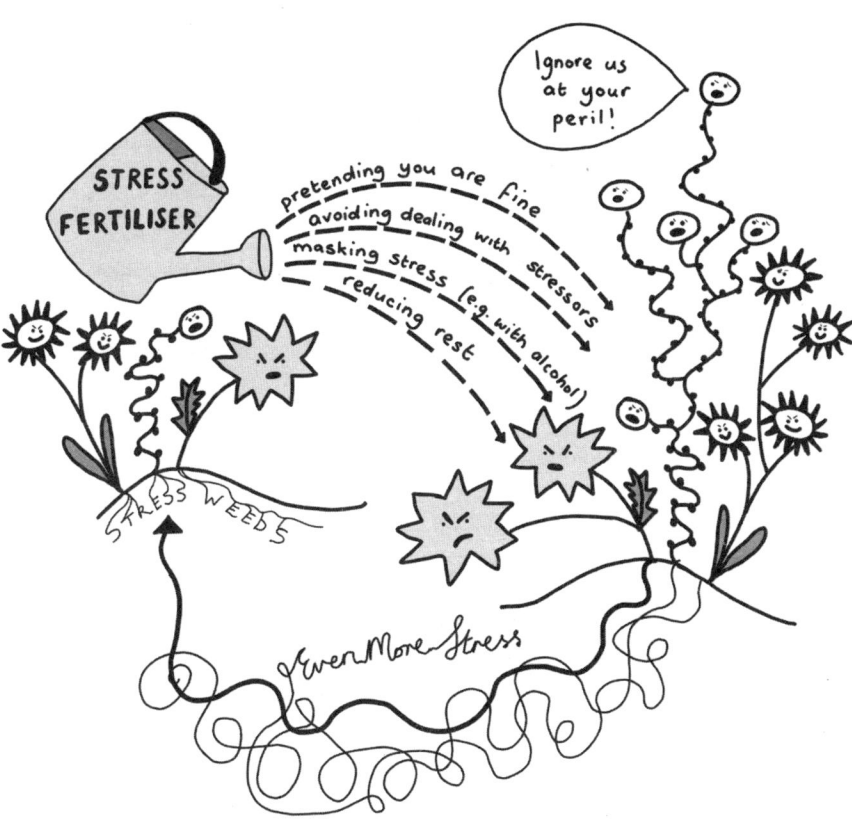

Anti-burnout Exercise 6: Weed suppression and prevention

There are multiple ways you can fertilize your stress weeds, through what you do, what you don't do and what you think. These things create more stress and/or extinguish opportunities to reduce it. Think about the ways you make your stress grow. Some of the common ways include:

- Avoidance: you might avoid tackling problems or speaking to people about how you feel, or even deny to yourself you are stressed.

> - How you talk to and treat yourself – do you nurture yourself or take a big metaphorical stick and beat yourself up?
> - Substance and alcohol use
> - Eating less healthily, irregularly or too much or too little
> - Technology use
> - Not seeing friends
> - Not taking breaks from work
>
> Use the image on page 79 to think about the factors that feed your stress weed and create a vicious cycle.
>
> Now think about how you can create a cycle to suppress your stress weeds, e.g. ways to create a helpful pattern that reduces the weeds.

Antidotes to stress: Giving the 'rest and digest' response the credit it deserves

Remember the two important parts of the stress responses we need to keep us healthy:

1) Ramping up or switching on via the sympathetic nervous system.

2) Dimming down and switching off via the parasympathetic nervous system.

Too often we overlook and neglect the second part (we'll go into some of the reasons why in the next few chapters). This means that many of us stay in stress mode for too long, because we don't give enough credit to or value the second part of the stress cycle, which is critical for keeping us healthy: our rest and digest system. This anti-burnout exercise is designed to give the second part of the stress cycle the attention, credit and value it deserves both proactively and when we notice we are stressed.

In my clinical work I use an analogy of cycling up and down a hill to think about the stress cycle. It's simple, yet it captures exactly what we need to do to manage stress, but what we so often overlook. We need to notice we are going up the stress hill and then make sure we come down it again to recover. If we keep going uphill for too long, we use too much energy and deplete ourselves. To complete our stress (bi)cycle route, we have to shift gear and put the brakes on in some way, to switch off the stress response, to move into recovery mode and ensure we activate our parasympathetic nervous system. Using this idea can help make shifting gear to go downhill on the stress cycle a regular and normal part of our routine.

This exercise is about reactively noticing stress/high demand and completing the cycle route. However, we can also ensure we proactively give the 'rest and digest' response the credit it deserves during the day to help us stay healthy, too. While you are completing this exercise, think about how you can build the activities that shift your gear into downhill mode into your day on a regular basis, as they will help protect you from burnout.

Anti-burnout Exercise 7: Complete your stress (bi)cycle route

To stay healthy, we need to go uphill, but we also need the necessary brakes and recovery from that high-energy switched-on mode. I have found from my clinical work and personal experience that we often fail to do the second part of the stress cycle. It's taken me a mindset shift to overcome my tendency to keep on keeping on. There are many ways we can do this, and how you complete your stress cycle will be personal to you and will shift according to your energy and needs. Some simple ways include:

- Taking good-quality breaks.
- Doing things that get you in the flow state.
- Doing things you enjoy that relax you or make you feel good.
- Having routines that mark a separation between work and rest.

There are some ideas in the image opposite, too. Note what helps you shift into downhill mode, and how you can remind yourself to do this.

Under pressure

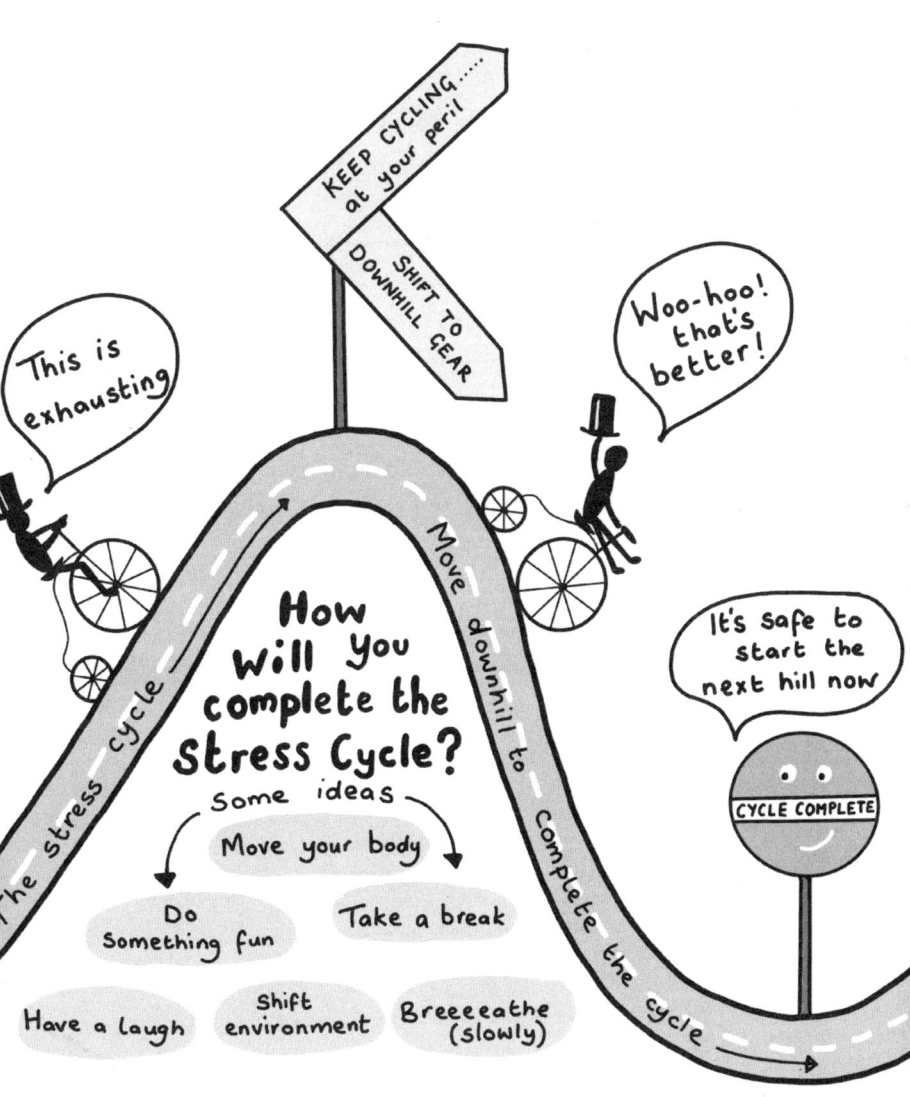

Anti-burnout takeaways:

- Stress can be thought of as our experience of how our body responds to stressors.
- It is important to understand your signs of stress to help you notice when you are stressed.
- Looking at your level of stress can help you understand how to manage it.
- If demands outweigh capacity, it can lead to overwhelm. The capacity cup can help you notice and manage your capacity.
- The body stress response is a critical function that helps us through life. Our body is designed to recover from stress.
- Chronic stress is when you experience too much stress or high levels of stress for too long, with no chance to recover. This is detrimental to your physical and mental health and can lead to burnout.
- Recognizing whether your coping strategies help or contribute to your stress can help you break this pattern.
- Remembering to complete the stress cycle route (engage your 'rest and digest' system) – by ensuring you shift gear, put the brakes on and go downhill when you experience stress – can help you manage stress.

Chapter 4
Beliefs and burnout

There's a critical piece of the stress puzzle I have missed out so far, and that's our thoughts. Whether we find something stressful or not is, to some extent, mediated by the thoughts we have about the event. Thoughts can also be a stressor, for example if we are constantly nasty to ourselves (we'll come back to this later), it sets off our body stress responses and we experience more stress. But thoughts are more than just mediators of stress – they are with us throughout our life as the constant chatter or images in our head telling us what to do or what not to do; guiding, disrupting, supporting, berating, judging or evaluating us. They can appear automatically or be carefully constructed. They can whisper or shout at us. They influence what we do and how we feel. But this is a two-way interaction: what's going on can also influence our thoughts – the content and nature can shift dependent on how we feel. But where do thoughts derive from? To understand this, let's look at my current thoughts.

My automatic thoughts were telling me to keep going, push through and get this chapter done. But now my current thoughts are consciously shouting at me, 'It's time to take a break before you start this chapter, Emma!' Such a simple statement, so why is it so hard for me to implement and why did my brain automatically tell me different? To understand this, we have to go below the thoughts to reach our belief systems, which can drive not only our thoughts but also our perception of and interactions with the world.

What are beliefs?

We can think of beliefs as constructs that help our brain to shape, filter and understand the complex information constantly coming through our perceptions. Linked associations between information in our brain create schemas, or mental maps, which provide a quick, easy guide for us to understand the vast amount of information coming at us. Effectively, they are a shortcut to help us understand the world at a glance. Consider the London Underground map (or the equivalent for other cities): a simplified guide that helps us get our bearings quickly and make sense, at a glance, of a complex transport system. It is a structured framework that provides an organized way of perceiving, understanding and responding to complex information. Without these quick guides to the world, we would be overwhelmed and unable to make sense of the shapes, sounds, objects and vast amount of information. Not only do such maps help us understand the world, but they also influence what we see, what we experience and how we think, respond and behave. But just like maps, our beliefs sometimes become outdated and, therefore, are unhelpful to us.

HOW DO BELIEFS BUILD IN OUR BRAIN?

Where do our beliefs come from? How do our brains construct these quick guides that play such a powerful influence on how us humans see and interact with the world? Like our brain predictions, these beliefs are shaped and constructed through our experiences of the world. The environments we live in shape our beliefs directly and indirectly, through the statements we have been told and the behaviours we have observed.

Our childhood experience is critical in shaping these beliefs, as our childhood brain is developing rapidly and creating the structures and connections that take us through life. Our beliefs are designed to tell us how the world will and should respond, what is safe, who we are and our place in the world. Those closest to us – parents, caregivers, family and friends – usually have a critical role in shaping our beliefs, through what they do and what they say (often transmitting their own belief systems through generations).

However, there are many other influences on our belief systems – they are shaped by various social, political, cultural and economic factors. All the environments we exist in give us messages, including home, school, work and social circles. The messages we are given through television, social media, newspapers, books or wherever you get your information from shapes our beliefs. The people we observe – leaders, politicians and public figures – and the messages they give us can have pivotal roles in shaping our beliefs. If we think about factors that might have shaped belief systems throughout history, they may include religious, political, industrial, scientific and medical systems.

Let's think about some important types of beliefs that shape us and the world in which we live. These include beliefs about sex roles, mental health and emotions, cultures and groups of people, children and parenting, how humans should live and what matters to us. In our own brain we construct beliefs around ourselves (who we are as people) others (individuals and groups) and the external world. These beliefs influence how we see and respond to ourselves, the world and people around us.

How belief systems impact life

Beliefs influence everything we do, whether we are aware of them consciously or not. But like all helpful brain functions (and just like stress), they can become unhelpful to us. Beliefs can lead to bias and stigma towards ourselves and others. They can stop us doing things that would be helpful (just look at my automatic thoughts about writing this chapter – what did they tell you about my beliefs?), they make us do things we don't want to and can lead us to respond to challenges in unhelpful ways. Beliefs about ourselves can be particularly harsh, and we can become our own bully. We often apply beliefs to ourselves that wouldn't even cross our mind with other people. Our beliefs can lead to our brain only filtering in information that confirms them, such as a negative view of ourselves.

BELIEF-SHIFTING

Shifting beliefs is critical to changing harmful and unhelpful thoughts and behaviours. It's part of how we improve our mental health, change our behaviour, treat ourselves and others better, and reduce stigma and discrimination. I don't think its overly dramatic to say it's how we create a better world.

The good thing is that our beliefs are shifting all the time. I am not the same psychologist (or person) I was twenty years ago, because my beliefs have shifted with my new experiences, learning and interactions. I now respond and see the world differently compared to my past self. You will not be the same person for your whole life either; you are in a constant state

Beliefs and burnout

of change, your brain is constantly creating new connections between the 86 billion or so neurons that make up its information highway and construct your internal belief 'maps'.

Belief change can be as simple as a conversation, learning new information, reading a book, hearing someone else's perspective, watching a TV show, travelling to a different country or even meeting someone new. These help our brain evolve and create new neural networks that shift our belief systems from what we know into something different (hopefully something more helpful, but not always). This is constantly happening and will hopefully happen when you read this chapter. BUT there is a BIG but.

Our beliefs are powerful, sneaky things that tend to make us see what we already believe. They filter the world so we receive information that confirms what we know, thereby strengthening those networks in our brain.[1] The self-perpetuating nature of beliefs makes them notoriously hard to shift. They might become entrenched for a number of reasons, for instance if:

- they have been particularly strong or repeated messages;
- they were built in childhood, when the brain is particularly vulnerable;
- we have had constantly confirmatory experiences;
- we haven't been exposed to other possible beliefs.

We are often not even aware these beliefs are there or how they impact on us. Our beliefs sit insidiously in our brain, not always revealing or exposing themselves, affecting how we think and behave without our awareness. It is for this very reason that unconscious bias occurs.

THE NEGATIVITY BIAS STRIKES AGAIN

Remember how our brain has a highly negative bias? This negative bias is needed to survive in this unpredictable world, and guess what that means? Negative beliefs are even more powerful and insidious – a dangerous combination that means they have a strong influence, are self-perpetuating and are difficult to shift.

There's another reason these negative beliefs are harder to kick, and to explain that, we are back to my old friend Shane, aka shame. We often feel shameful about what our negative beliefs tell us, which means we want to keep them hidden, to protect ourselves. But this has the opposite effect to that intended. Hiding them means we can't open them up to other perspectives; we are unable to filter in or openly receive contradictory information. We can't expose them to the light, where they can be tackled and shifted. Keeping these shameful beliefs hidden feels safe but means they exponentially self-perpetuate, and strengthen the networks throughout our brain, exerting even stronger influences on how we view and interact with the world.

The good news is that it's possible to change them. By understanding our underground networks of beliefs and bringing them out in the open for critique, we can take action to shift them.

One last word of warning. Beliefs are a bit like Voldemort – they have the power to grow back even when we think they are vanquished. Although we consciously say and think we believe one thing, lurking negative beliefs try to pull us back into their grip, making us see information and drive behaviours that enable them to take control again (just look at my initial thoughts at the start of this chapter, for example).

Old unhelpful beliefs are particularly likely to resurface when our brain is depleted – the hallmark of a burnout brain. We thought we'd forgotten them, laid them to rest, left them in the past where they belonged, but they were only resting, waiting to re-emerge and gather strength again when our resources and defences were down, so they could strike back with a powerful force that beats our burnout brain into oblivion.

Beliefs and burnout

But why do our beliefs matter for burnout? Well, as we've seen, beliefs matter for everything we do, so they matter for burnout too. You may have spotted that I've already been talking about my beliefs that contributed to my burnout. These beliefs are critical branches in my burnout tree (see page 42). Beliefs drive behaviours that contribute to burnout and can make you less likely to do the things to help you recover. In addition, when we are depleted through burnout, the Voldemorts of our brain are more likely to bounce back, taking control and exerting their sinister influence. When I work with burnout patients, identifying and shifting beliefs are at the heart of what we do to change burnout trajectories. We can also build beliefs that protect you from burnout – strengthening your burnout tree and helping you manage stress. Let's start with some of my beliefs that were critical to my burnout, before we move on to yours.

You may have spotted some clues to some of the beliefs that contributed to my burnout. Remember I said I never wanted to be dramatic? What does this tell us? It probably taps into beliefs about how I should display or share emotions, and possibly beliefs about how women should share emotions. Now let's get this straight, I don't consciously believe that we shouldn't show emotions – for goodness' sake, I'm a psychologist, I believe the opposite! However, they were commonly held beliefs as I grew up (and for many thousands of years beforehand[2] – hey, I told you that beliefs are notoriously hard to shift). But I have to face facts that these beliefs are in my grey matter somewhere and have created underground networks in my brain that are affecting my life, through my behaviour and attitudes. The fact that beliefs often lurk when we don't consciously think them is demonstrated well with research around unconscious bias. For example, very few of us would say we were racist, but research demonstrates many of us have racist beliefs working away in the depths of our brain – unconscious bias that influences the decision we make and behaviours we demonstrate. (See Pragya Agarwal's' book[3] for an overview of unconscious bias.)

One of my beliefs that I discovered during burnout and that surprised me was the belief that if I am not feeling stressed then I am not working hard enough. How ridiculous is that? However, when I tentatively voiced this in a meeting, it turns out this was a common belief in people working in the same healthcare system as I was.

Some of my unhelpful beliefs were outdated maps, helpful at other stages of my life but not under current circumstances. Some of these were Voldemort beliefs – shadows from the past that I no longer believe but that had re-emerged when I was depleted. And some of them I didn't even realize I had – I don't consciously believe them but they exist in my brain somewhere, exerting an unseen influence over my thoughts and actions. You will have the same. We are going to look at my top four countdown of burnout beliefs. Before we do, let's stop and think about your beliefs and how they might contribute to burnout.

Anti-burnout Exercise 8: Identifying unhelpful beliefs

What beliefs have you noticed about yourself that may contribute to burnout? It's important to note that they aren't necessarily unhelpful generally, but they may become unhelpful dependent on the situation you are in and the level of pressure you are under. Have you noticed beliefs that surface when you are feeling bad, or when your resources are depleted? If you are having trouble identifying your underground networks of beliefs, then notice what these prompts bring to mind for you:

- What messages were you given about yourself and the world as you were growing up?
- What were common beliefs about work, sex roles, emotions and mental health as you were growing up or in your culture?
- Are there any patterns of thoughts you have that are clues to your beliefs?
- What are your beliefs about:
    - success or achievement
    - being busy and productive
    - rest/relaxation/downtime
    - coping or struggling
    - emotions
- What do you tell yourself when you are feeling bad or your resources are depleted? This can give insight into your beliefs about yourself or emotions.
- Are there beliefs that you hold about yourself that you don't hold about other people?
- Have you noticed any underlying beliefs that surprise you, because you don't consciously believe them?

Burnout Belief 4: Life is a game of Donkey Kong: you will get THERE (if you just ... work hard enough)

Do you treat life like a game of Donkey Kong? Work hard enough, complete enough levels (possibly defeat a few big baddies) and you will get the reward at the end – you will arrive in the mythical land of THERE. This mythical 'there' is the idea we will complete life in some way, life will be sorted and we will be forever-happy, contented beings. For me the mythical 'there' was when I was able to breeze through any situation calmly with poise, with no self-doubt, feeling constantly in control of parenting, life, work (of course with a ZERO inbox) and having achieved the perfect work/life balance. For most people there is a mythical THERE in their life, an end point they are striving for. Maybe you think that once you reach that point you will feel constantly on top of things, you will be fully expert with not a touch of imposter, or feel fully adult and totally in charge of life. Fundamentally it boils down to some form of 'when I reach THERE I will master being a human and be in absolute control of the complex world and the stuff it throws at me.'

I can tell you that as I reach my fifties, at each point I feel I am almost THERE, the 'almost there rug' is pulled from beneath my feet and the end point vanishes. Sadly, although we might sometimes get there temporarily, or feel like we are nearly there, THERE is a slippery character. As soon as you are within touching distance, it slips from your fingers, to be seemingly just out of reach again. This means you have to work a bit harder, do more, gain more knowledge, get another promotion, buy just one more thing, or become more

Beliefs and burnout

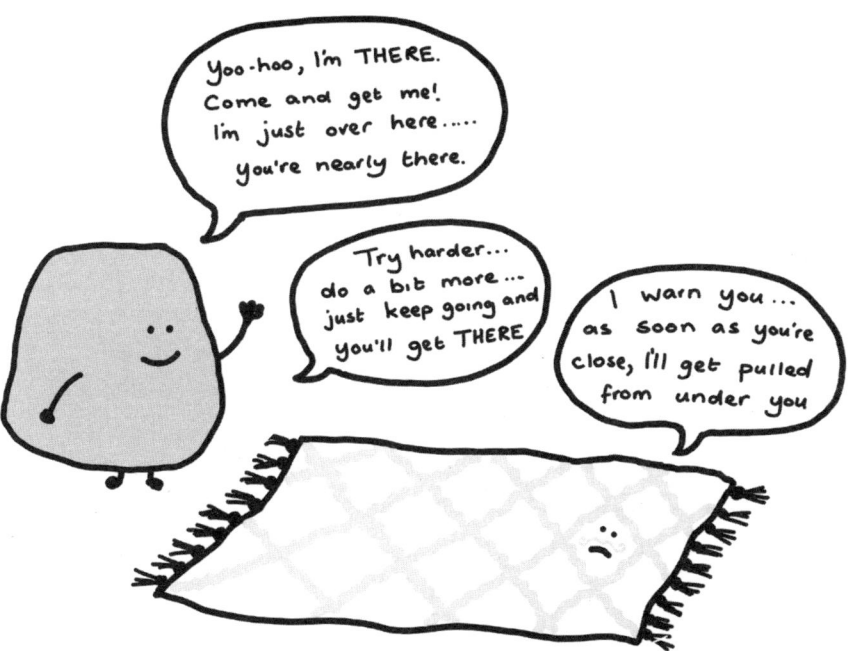

competent to get THERE again. THERE likes to make you think it is a tangible location that you can arrive at, so you are constantly striving, struggling, wishing, working, spending, trying to reach it and all it promises. It keeps you on the treadmill, trying to reach an unrealistic goal and making you feel like a failure for not getting THERE.

Of course, THERE does not exist; it's an illusion designed to make you think the messiness of life is something that you are responsible for, that you need to strive to overcome rather than learn to live with. At first this realization may feel demotivating, but ultimately, recognizing THERE is mythical can be freeing. You will never get rid of difficult emotions, fully master being human or solve all your problems, so you don't have to. None of us is perfect, always confident, happy and content or fully in control, so you don't have to be. Recognizing THERE is a tantalizing endpoint that doesn't exist means you can STOP the futile use of energy constantly trying to reach this mythical goal and instead direct energy towards achievable goals. You can celebrate NOW by starting imperfectly and doing the things that make you happy and feel good – you don't have to wait for the fireworks to happen when you complete the game.

Life (unfortunately) is not a Donkey Kong game, where we get to conquer the baddies and celebrate completion. We will constantly be going up and down and through the levels with complex emotions, new problems arising, feeling out of control at times and navigating the ups and downs thrown at us. Your job is not to conquer the messiness of life, your job is to learn to live with and navigate this as best you can.

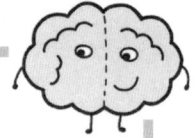

Brian the Brain reflections

- Where is your THERE you have been trying to reach?
- What would theoretically happen when you get THERE?
- Is this realistically achievable?
- Does this drive your behaviour in unhelpful ways?
- Are you blaming yourself for things that are just human?
- What can you accept instead of beating yourself up about?
- Where can you direct your energy instead of trying to get THERE?

Burnout Belief 3: Working 9-5 (then 5-9): productivity, achievement and rest

We have an unfortunate way of transmitting some of our own unhelpful beliefs to our children through what we say and do. I caught myself the other day telling my children not to be lazy (they were watching TV after a full day of school and sports). But I didn't stop there (have some empathy for me, I was in a bad mood). I then said, 'Imagine what you could have achieved with all the hours of TV you've watched - you could have practised your guitar and become an expert guitar player.' What message was I unwittingly telling my children? That they should be constantly productive and achieving. That rest was a waste of time and lazy, which is something bad. You should just keep going even when you feel tired or ill or depleted. Oh dear, and we wonder why people burn out ...

It's imperative that we look at beliefs about productivity, because they are intrinsically tied into how we work and use our time and whether we rest, or not. I cannot deny (as you have seen) that I have internalized messages about productivity and achievement, and these have led to behaviours that contributed to my burnout. For example, I remember saying: 'I rest by doing things.' Now, to some extent this is true, as actions like gardening and baking are inherently relaxing for me. But in reality, it meant I was always doing rather than taking time to relax. I share this not to shame myself, but to show how these beliefs show up and exert their influence over our behaviour, and lead to burnout.

It's interesting to think about where these beliefs come from and how they are entrenched in our societies and the messages we receive (which may differ across cultures). In her fascinating book *Exhausted,* Anna Katharina Schaffner[4] looks at the origins of cultural attitudes towards work and rest and how they affect our own attitudes and behaviour. She argues that these beliefs are intrinsically linked to capitalism, which developed alongside the Industrial Revolution. Our jobs have become part of our identity and we are constantly working, as we are always striving to have more, never satisfied with what we have. Religion, and more specifically the protestant work ethic, is also thought to have played a part, with busyness being seen as a virtue, and sloth as sinful. Schaffner shares the idea that wasting time was viewed as the biggest sin – and how many of us have internalized this idea? Currently, I see this belief being propagated further over social media all the time with productivity hacks, 5am wake-ups and optimization techniques being shared everywhere.

This push for productivity can lead to a sense of urgency and feeling we need to make the most of all our time, rushing and being busy constantly. You can only relax once you have achieved enough; rest is unproductive and not a good use of time. We can't stop or pause, as we can't spare the time; we need to do more and feel we have never done enough. We feel like we are wasting our time when ill or resting (or even ignore illness because we don't have time to deal with it – guilty as charged). Activities that should be relaxing become only worth it if we achieve or produce. Reading becomes worth it only for the gathering of information; exercise for the losing of weight. Our hobbies become levers to achieve rather than panaceas of stress, as they should be, thereby quashing the inherently relaxing qualities of these activities and rendering them as another thing to achieve on our 'to do' list.

Worst of all, we tie our busyness and achievements into our identity. Our achievements become the very definition of who we are and our worth. Resting can feel like a challenge to our identity – who are we when we are not busy or achieving?

We don't stop, because stopping, resting, pausing reduces our ability to produce, achieve, be successful, and ultimately makes us somehow a lesser human. This all leads to greater pressure and stress, adding weight to our tree's branches.

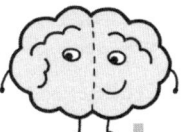

Brian the Brain reflections

- What are your beliefs about busyness/achievement/productivity?
- What are your beliefs about rest?
- Do you tie these factors into your identity?
- What do these beliefs make you do?
- What do these beliefs stop you doing?
- How do these beliefs increase your risk of burnout?

Burnout Belief 2: WHO AM I? (And what is this contingent on?)

I hate that request in an interview: 'Tell me about yourself.' But I'm going to say it to you now, as it taps into our identity, how we see and define ourselves. So, stop and think now – who are you? How would you describe yourself? How we view ourselves is critical, as our sense of self influences how we interact with the world. Life can sometimes pose challenges to our identity from which we need to adapt or rebuild. Burnout can leave you asking, who am I? But your 'who am I?' can contribute to burnout in the very first place.

Many of us have a fundamentally negative views of ourselves – we are not good enough (or just not enough), in some way inadequate, and other people are all doing far better than us. Through my clinical work, I have commonly heard people say they are useless, a waste of space, will never do anything good, that nobody likes them (believe me, these are common beliefs linked to mental health difficulties). Or we believe we are only good enough or worthwhile if we perform, behave or achieve in a particular way, meaning our identity is enmeshed with these very factors. This means that our worth is contingent on certain factors such as getting THERE (we already know that's impossible), success, achievement, coping, not feeling bad, productivity or how other people view us. This creates a fragile identity and worth which are always on shaky ground because these factors are very difficult, or impossible, to maintain as constants in our lives. It can also mean we work hard to achieve these things, using our energy to maintain our identity through impossible means – constant achievement, perfection (see opposite), success and keeping people happy. And when this fails (because it will), it causes greater stress and has a greater impact. Because it's not just about not achieving, not being successful or not being liked – it's a fundamental reflection and indictment on who we are as a person. It means we are a worthless, rubbish human.

Brian the Brain reflections

- How would you describe yourself?
- What positive beliefs do you have about yourself?
- What does your inner critic say to you? (This can be an indication of your negative beliefs about yourself.)*
- Is your worth contingent on certain factors? What are they?

---

* If your beliefs are very critical and impacting on you negatively (how you feel or what you do) then it is worth considering addressing this through psychological intervention/therapy.

Burnout Belief 1: The perfect storm

Our beliefs, of course, don't sit in separate segments in our brains; they all intermingle in that underground map to create our view of the world. Something that is influential across all the previous burnout beliefs is our relationship to failure and, conversely, our idea of what 'good enough' means. To many of us, the only 'good enough' is perfection, and failure is a damning indictment on who we are as a person. Perfection can be a mythical THERE, something we strive to achieve to our detriment, because we will work harder, push ourselves further and never stop in order to pursue this unobtainable and mythical perfection. If we believe we should be perfect, then anything but (yes, that's nearly everything) is a significant challenge to our identity - anything less than perfect can feel unacceptable, abominable, devastating. Therefore, we work harder, we maintain impossible standards, are in constant fear of getting something wrong, feel like an imposter, or avoid things or procrastinate, because we are fearful the outcome won't meet our impossible standards (spoiler: it won't). No wonder the pursuit of perfection is stressful, and research tells us perfectionism is one of those branches that adds to the load and leads to burnout.[5]

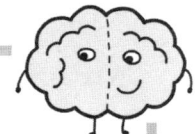

Brian the Brain reflections

- Do you feel you always have to achieve perfection?
- What do you tell yourself if you don't achieve perfection?
- What are your beliefs about failure?
- What do you tell yourself if you feel like you have failed?
- How do these beliefs impact on what you do/how you feel?

Other burnout beliefs

Of course, these are not the only beliefs that contribute to burnout. There are as many flavours of beliefs as ice cream (we can even have beliefs about ice cream!). Other beliefs that I believe (yes, we can even have beliefs about beliefs!) are important, through my clinical work and research, include those about:

- Emotions and mental health
- Being independent and what it means to seek support
- Tending to our own needs
- Gender roles
- Definitions of success

We'll look at some of these in more detail as we go through the book. There may be others too that you recognize have been important branches in your tree, mingling with your life and stressors to increase your risk of burnout. Beliefs are often tucked away deep in our brain and opening them up can be difficult – if you are noticing very negative beliefs about yourself, the world or other people, and/or recognize these have arisen from very difficult experiences or trauma, then it is worth considering whether you need to tackle these in therapy.

UNDOING THE MESSAGING

How do we allow ourselves to be imperfect humans who will fail? How do we extricate the need for perfection from our identity, and how can we shift failure to be just part of life rather than a fundamental reflection on who we are as person? How do we reshape our old, outdated beliefs and build a set of beliefs that serve us, and in which we truly believe?

It starts with understanding our beliefs and knowing how they influence us and our view of the world. It's about noticing

Beliefs and burnout

when they show up and what they make us see and do, and what they stop us from doing. You can use the reflections earlier to help with this. You can then start to recognize and empathize with your old beliefs, and where they came from, while acknowledging they no longer serve you. You can start to write yourself a new set of beliefs. You can open your brain to experiences and ideas that contradict and shift your beliefs, helping you to develop new ones. Opening up to people, sharing your stories and hearing other people's stories, is powerful too – it stops your own stories self-perpetuating via shame, validates and normalizes your messy human experience and connects with others. I have included a range of resources (see Further Reading, page 306) that I have found helpful to tackle these top four burnout beliefs.

Beliefs can be hard to shift, especially those ingrained negative ones that have really taken hold of our brain's neuronal networks; but that doesn't mean we shouldn't take action to tackle them and build beliefs that we want to live our lives by.

To do this, let's come back to my kids. It can be helpful to reframe beliefs by thinking about what message you *do* really want to share or live by. I have tried my hardest to undo some of the messaging imbued in my brain, by thinking about what messaging I want to pass on to my kids and demonstrating healthier beliefs to them through my action and words. For example, instead of berating them for wasting their time when watching TV, I emphasize the important of rest and downtime, both through what I say and what I do. Our new beliefs might not initially override those old ingrained ones, but they can start to shift them and gradually build, so you can live your life by them. I first came across the idea of a personal manifesto from Lauren Currie, who runs UPFRONT, an organization on a mission to upskill women, and I think it's the perfect way to reset your beliefs and build new ones you want to live your life around. There's something powerful about setting your own manifestos and thereby beliefs, rather than letting the world and other people build them for you.

Anti-burnout Exercise 9: Building your OWN manifesto

1. Old belief that no longer serves you

Note down an old, unhelpful belief and how it influences your behaviour/shows up in your life.

2. The new belief you want to live your life by

Note a more helpful belief you would like to replace this with.

3. How will you cultivate this new belief?

What will you do to help this belief guide your life? It could be new habits, routines or repeating affirmations.

Old belief that no longer serves me	The new belief I want to live my life by	How will I cultivate this new belief?

Anti-burnout takeaways

- Beliefs are structures stored in our brain about how the world operates. They influence how we think, what we see, what we do and how we interact with the world.
- Some beliefs can be part of the burnout tree. They can contribute to burnout as they can lead us to think in ways, interpret things and do things that create or increase our stress.
- Even when we don't consciously think these things, we can have beliefs that influence our behaviour which have developed as a result of the context and cultures in which we exist.
- Outdated negative beliefs can start to influence us again when we are depleted.
- Some beliefs that can contribute to burnout are beliefs about:
  - Arriving at a mythical THERE
  - Productivity and achievement
  - How we view ourselves
  - Failure and perfection
- Understanding your beliefs can help you understand how they influence your behaviour and to untangle them from your brain.
- Building a personal manifesto can help you set your own beliefs that guide you through life.

Chapter 5
Let's get physical, and emotional

Britney told us all about toxic stress, now it's over to Olivia Newton-John to look at another key element of an anti-burnout manifesto: looking after our physical and emotional needs. So, join me and Olivia in singing, 'Let's get physical (and emotional)'!

One of the main jobs of the brain is to predictively manage our body budget, deciding where, when and how to spend resources to keep things running smoothly. Your brain is constantly listening to your body's signals and predicting your energy needs in order to budget the resources your body needs to function, stay healthy and keep your energy in balance. To do this, your body and brain are speaking to each other all the time, giving signals that are indicators of our needs – and they want you to listen.

Through the process of interoception, your clever brain is constantly making sense of the internal information coming at you. We make sense of the signals by giving them a name – sadness, hunger, illness, stress, tiredness – and processing the information tells us what we need to do. For example:

- Growling stomach = hungry = eat
- Weariness = lack of energy = rest

Let's get physical, and emotional

- Tightening muscles = something is stressful = deal with the stressor
- Uneasy feeling in a meeting = something is not meeting your values = raise a question
- Low and lethargic = being sad = need support
- Starting to feel a bit bleurgh = coming down with something = rest and recuperate
- Feeling more bleurgh = red alert = see a doctor

But it's not just about specific signals; your brain also tries to summarize a lot of the data to give a general sense of the state of your body budget and how full or depleted it is. This summary, called affect, is a clever mechanism designed to give you information about your overall needs so you can respond. 'Body budget' is a term coined by psychologist Lisa Feldman-Barrett, based on her research, to describe the level of resources your body currently has, which is indicated by that general sense of how you feel (affect). She tells us:

Like a financial budget, a body budget can run a deficit, and over the long term, a bankrupt body budget results in illness.

Other animals don't question these signals, they just respond to them. However, humans are complex and have a brain that analyzes, questions, believes, debates and overrides this information. As a result, we can become our own worst enemies and make the seemingly simple task of responding to our body signals a lot harder than it needs to be, resulting in a bankrupt body budget and greater risk of burnout.

The Anti-Burnout Book

Why we battle our body signals

To begin making sense of why we often don't listen to or respond to the needs our body is highlighting, let's travel back to the north of Scotland in the 1980s, more specifically to the school dining hall of beige plastic stools and equally beige meals. Woe betide those who didn't eat their meals: the fierce dinner ladies stood over the slop bucket and sent you back to your seat if you hadn't eaten enough. I remember one particularly vivid occasion when delightfully grey steak and kidney was served – it was rank. I tried in vain to hide it under my napkin and dispose of it into the slop bucket but was sent back. On the third failed attempt, I remember being told, 'There's starving children in the world and you, little lady, have the audacity to not eat the food you are given.' With the beady eye of the dinner lady now fixed on me, I had no choice but to eat the grey slop. I felt sick for the rest of the day (in fact, I still feel sick at the thought of it) and have never eaten steak and kidney since. The message? 'Don't listen to your body telling you this is rank.' When food was semi-decent, the message was: 'Don't listen to your body when it is full.' Force yourself to eat it, despite what your body is telling you. If you don't, you are doing something wrong and should be ashamed of yourself.

The messaging was around other body signals too – one day I had to finish all my free school milk and my friend's, because she hated milk (remember, we HAD to drink it). Afterwards, bursting, I asked to go to the toilet in class but was told I should be able to hold it in until the end of class. So I did what I was told to do and held it in, until sadly I couldn't anymore and Darren put his hand up and said, 'Miss, miss! Someone's peed on the floor!' Despite the fact I had been surreptitiously trying to hide it with my bag, it was obvious who the pee belonged to.

Let's get physical, and emotional

I still remember the shame, over forty years later, of having to change into someone else's blue gym knickers from the grubby spare kit box. That is now an amusing family story, and an unfortunate personal core memory. However, while my stories are useful to make my kids laugh, through my clinical work I have heard many sad stories about how we have been told to suppress our body's indicators of our needs. The message is that instead of listening to our body's signals we need to override them with what we think we should be doing. This leads to the inevitable outcome that instead of responding to our needs, we learn to ignore, override, mask, suppress or even start to feel ashamed of them.

The reasons why we don't respond to body signals link to messages about productivity and achievement, how they are valued, and, conversely, to messages we may have received about rest and taking time off. I remember there being pride in our family about having never taken a day off work (I really think they should have). We all have our own personal experiences of messages and how these impacted on us. Our body and brain learn to adapt and survive in the environment in which they exist, which might mean that we adapted to align with directly received or cultural messages. However, for some people, suppressing needs or emotions may have been a necessary survival mechanism that kept them safe in the situation they were in but are no longer helpful longer term.

Whatever the reason for these learned behaviours – such as ignoring or masking our needs – it is important to recognize when they no longer serve us, because if we don't respond to our body when it's shouting about its needs, ultimately this leads to depletion.

> **Brian the Brain reflections**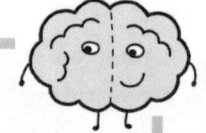
>
> - How are you at responding to your body signals?
> - Are there times you ignore or suppress these signals?
> - Are there signals you could get better at responding to?
> - What could you do to help you notice and respond to your body signals?

Emotions as body signals

Now let's shift our attention to emotions. Emotions are complex little (or sometimes big) things. I've spoken about the science of emotion in my previous book,[1] so we won't go into the full scientific detail here (it is fascinating – if you want to find out more, see page 306). At this point, it's enough to say that emotions are also bodily signals – information that indicates our needs – in the same way that hunger, sleepiness or needing to pee do. It's just that we tend to categorize them differently and have an extra layer of complexity around how we think about them, linked to thousands of years of long-held beliefs about emotions and the mind/body dichotomy. This means they often come with an extra-large dollop of unhelpful messaging and unhelpful beliefs, which – yes, you guessed it – leads to unhelpful behaviour around our emotions, and sometimes leads us to failing to notice them at all!

The long-held beliefs go something like this (I'm trying to capture a thousand years of history in a sentence here): we should only feel specific emotions; some emotions are bad; some are bad depending on your sex; and struggling or letting bad emotions overwhelm you is a personal failure or weakness.

Hmmm, I wonder why there is still stigma around emotions and mental health? We ain't going to shift those long-held thousand-years of beliefs overnight, or even over a decade. It's a good and worthy fight but it will take time, as a culture and for yourself, so be patient.

Emotions are a fundamental part of our brain functioning. They are neither rational nor irrational, and they are linked to nearly everything we do; learning, memory, attention, decision-making and forming bonds with others. Learning to understand that we can't extricate how we feel from our lives and that emotions are not something to override or overcome but something to learn about and understand, can enable us to use these body signals to help guide us through life instead of battling them. Ultimately, emotions are body signals too, information we can use to indicate our needs and manage our body budget. But we often have a lot of catching up to do in updating powerful societal beliefs and messaging about emotions and mental health before we can do this.

BATTLING OUR EMOTION SIGNALS

Let's think about how the messaging and beliefs about emotions plays out in our day to day lives. To do this, let's return to 1980s Scotland to help understand my insidious belief about being dramatic. Why do I think I am being dramatic when I am upset, and what does that lead to? I remember people being told not to be silly when they were crying or not to be a baby when they had a big emotional reaction. I also remember trying my hardest to stop crying on numerous occasions – I was not a crier (and hence not dramatic), and I was for some reason very proud of this. I had imbued some cultural attitudes, and no doubt received messages, that emotions should not be demonstrative and were something to be masked or kept within.

It's not just me who received these messages. They come hard and fast at many of us throughout life, through the stigmas around mental health and displaying difficult emotions: 'Stop crying, people will see you,' 'Don't be so dramatic!' (there, spot my belief). We turn these old, unscientifically supported and outdated beliefs about mental health and emotions into self-stigma. Through my clinical work I see this type of internalized stigma all the time. People feel ashamed because they feel bad and think they shouldn't talk about how they feel. We believe that other people would 'cope' better and berate ourselves for not battling through, and we view feeling bad as a personal failure or a sign of weakness.

We all know already what this messaging leads to: we suppress, mask, hide, try to control, bat away or don't even notice our emotions.

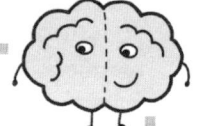

Brian the Brain reflections

- How are you at responding to your emotion body signals?
- Are there times when you ignore these signals?
- What beliefs around emotions stop you responding to these signals? What messages did you receive about having/showing emotions as you were growing up?
- Are there emotion signals you could get better at responding to?
- What could you do to help you notice and respond to your emotion body signals?

Your body budget and burnout

Ironically, the very emotion and body signals we're trying to push away benefit from being noticed, validated, spoken about and attended to. And guess what happens when we do push them way? It creates and amplifies stress through multiple mechanisms. Firstly, the very act of holding these feelings in (like me trying my hardest not to cry) is physiologically stressful for the body. Secondly, negating how we feel means we can't use these signals to take action or attend to our needs. As a result, we fail to recognize or seek support for issues and instead they fester or worsen (like my burnout) because we don't take action to shift their course. We can even add a third layer of stress by criticizing ourselves for how we feel, which stresses our body even further. We battle our body's signals and fail to top up our resources when it is telling us to, so our body budget falls into the red, becoming chronically overdrawn and depleted.

And yes, you've guessed it correctly – ignoring these emotional and physical signals is a superfast highway to burnout. Even when your body is shouting at you 'TAKE ACTION! STOP! REST! REFUEL! FOR GOODNESS' SAKE JUST PEE!' you keep on going. Eventually your brain and body give up, figuring out that you are not going to listen. They don't have the energy to shout anymore, and so adapt into a chronic stress mode, where your body budget is constantly running on empty, the predictions your brain is making are way off-course and even the signals, ignored for so long, have gone awry. I sometimes hear people in burnout say they can no longer trust their bodies, but I would flip this around. Your body can no longer trust you to respond or tend to its needs so it has given up trying – it's feeling hopeless and malfunctioning because not only have you not given it the annual MOT, but you have also failed to keep it topped up with even the very basic resources it needs to function on a day-to-day basis.

Let's give our body and emotion signals the attention they deserve to help us stay healthy. Sometimes we may need to tackle our belligerent beliefs to let us do this, and if this is the case for you, use Exercise 9 on page 104 to help with this. It's time to do this, so you can join the anti-burnout gang!

Anti-burnout Exercise 10: Managing your body budget

Just like your bank account, you need to keep an eye on your body budget and know your own balance. Regularly checking in on your budget can help you respond effectively. Are you flush and bounding with energy? Do you need a top-up? Are you seriously depleted?

You can keep your body budget in balance by managing deposits and withdrawals. You need to keep a regular eye on your balance to make sure you don't become overdrawn. You can top up proactively or when you notice your body budget units are becoming depleted, and you can manage withdrawals (though not all will be within your control).

Use the image opposite to:

1. Think about the state your body budget account is in currently. Does it need deposits to top it up? Doing this regularly can help you tune into your needs while keeping a healthy budget.

Let's get physical, and emotional

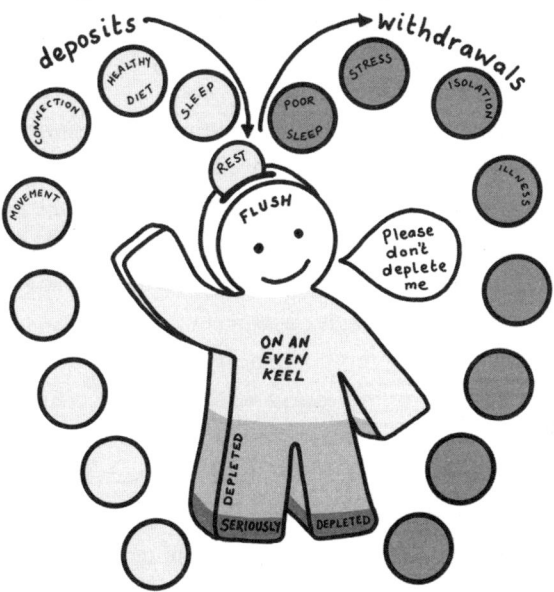

Where is your body budget?
Do you need to make any deposits?
What else creates deposits for you?

2. Think about what creates deposits of body budget units for you. Be wary that sometimes we make false deposits. These only mask your depletion temporarily and actually deplete you further (coffee was my crutch during burnout, but in reality it just gave me a temporary boost that masked my overall depletion).
3. Now think about what creates withdrawals of body budget units.
4. To become anti-burnout, you need to regularly manage your body budget to ensure it isn't depleted

> for too long or becomes overdrawn. Do this by monitoring the balance and considering whether you need to manage withdrawals or add deposits.
>
> Please note: If your budget has been sitting on empty or overdrawn for a long time, then it takes special measures to bring it back into the normal body budget scale. Consider this like being bankrupt (i.e. burned out). Yes, you can recover, but this is not like a normal bank account that you can keep in balance with quick deposits and withdrawals. When your body budget is bankrupt, it needs special measures to top it up and these require time and patience. It has been shown that it can take months or sometimes even years for your body to recover[2] – you might need time off to seriously look at your output and/or redesign your energy use drastically, to even get you back onto the normal body budget scale. We look at this further in Chapter 11.

Emotions as data

Okay, over to your emotions. Remember, we have to overcome thousands of years of powerful messaging here. This will likely be a gradual process to shift our beliefs about emotions, but it's a good fight worth having. The research tells us that if you learn to understand your emotions better, use the data effectively and respond helpfully to what the emotions are signalling, this is linked to better physical and mental health,[3] better wellbeing,[4] better relationship quality,[5] parenting and children's emotional understanding,[6] better responses to stress,[7] improved workplaces[8] and I'm not being dramatic when I say it builds a better world. Oh, and let's not overlook that

Let's get physical, and emotional

learning to respond to our emotions is even linked to how long we get to live on this beautiful, complex, messy planet of ours (your belligerent beliefs may be telling you not to believe me, but there is science that supports this[9]). So, while it might be effortful, it's certainly worthwhile.

Emotions are body signals we label with emotion words. Okay, the science is a bit more complex than that, but getting to know your emotions is the same as noticing you are hungry, thirsty or need to sleep. Emotions are just different labels we use to describe different body feelings.[10]

This might be more difficult than noticing other body feelings for a number of reasons: emotions are more subtle, complex and subjective, and they are linked to our language and culture. And of course, we've been telling ourselves for millennia or more that we should push these away, not feel a particular way or just not feel at all. This means that we find emotions harder to notice, understand and use as information to inform and guide our lives.

As children, learning to understand emotions is a skill we learn (or don't, as the case may be), which usually involves more complex cognition and language development to support it than noticing other body functions. For many adults, including Scottish ones that grew up in the 1980s, this just wasn't something we learned, and in fact it was something many of us intentionally tried to squish into oblivion. This means that many adults still have this skill to learn.

These skills are not just about noticing emotion but also more finely tuning our understanding of them, as well as changing our beliefs about them, our relationship with them and how we respond to them. An important part of psychological treatment and therapy can be learning to feel, because if we don't notice these emotions in the first the place, we can't do any of the fine tuning, so that's where we start with the next exercise.

The Anti-Burnout Book

Anti-burnout Exercise 11: What's the weather in your head?

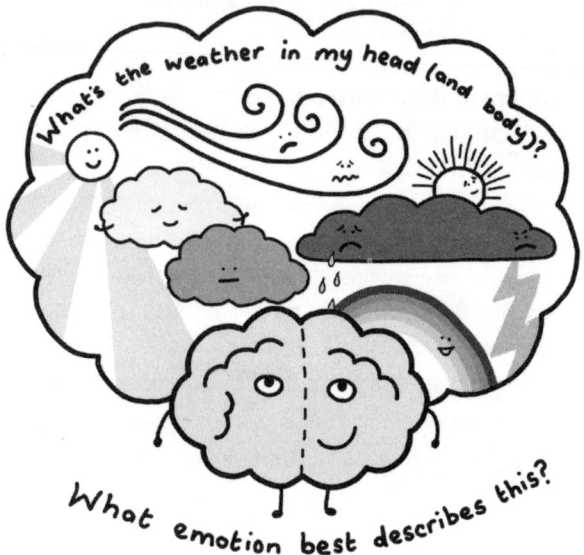

- What is your current weather? Describe your current body signals and how you are generally feeling.
- What is the best description that explains this weather? Pick an emotion that best describes how you feel.
- What is this weather telling you about your needs?
- What is this weather telling you about the situation you are in?
- Are there ways you are making the weather worse?
- What do you need to do (if anything) in response to this weather?

The best way to become anti-burnout is to not just respond to big emotions but also to stop, notice and think about the weather in your head (your emotions); to listen regularly to your body; and to know how you can understand and respond helpfully. This can take work if it's a skill you have never developed – see Further Reading on page 306 to explore more.

Anti-burnout takeaways

- To be anti-burnout we need to notice our body signals, recognize what they are saying about our needs and respond to them.
- This is about noticing and responding to our physical needs, such as tiredness, hunger and thirst.
- It is also about noting and responding to the body signals that indicate our emotional needs.
- Many of us have learned to mask, suppress or not respond to our body signals. This is even more pronounced for emotions, where long-term beliefs can lead us to bottle up, mask and suppress our emotions.
- Not responding to our physical or emotional body signals has a double impact: ignoring them means we don't attend to our needs and therefore don't manage stress or other body needs. In addition, suppressing or ignoring these signals is a stressful process in itself.
- Our beliefs about emotions often mean we neglect or ignore them. We may need to shift our beliefs in order to be able to respond to our body signals helpfully.
- We can learn to notice and respond to specific signals, such as emotions, pain, hunger and thirst.
- We can also learn to understand our overall body budget and keep it topped up regularly so we don't become depleted, which can contribute to burnout.

Chapter 6
Making work work for you: Let's take a look at your day job

Ah, work, that place where we spend most of our daily hours. That place we have been aiming towards all our lives. That place where we achieve purpose, success, fulfilment or at least enough money to live. That place where we feel supported by the wonderful team around us. That place where we spend nearly as much time with our colleagues as our family. That place of never-ending demand with no end to the 'to do' list. That place that you can no longer switch off from, as work and life merge into a blended whole. That side-hustle that was supposed to give you freedom but now has become a bind that you want to extricate yourself from. That place where you know your colleague doing the same job gets paid more. That place that causes stress, stress and more stress. That place where power-hungry managers exert their authority over you. That place where you deal with difficult emotions, stress and trauma daily and are expected to just get on with it. That place where you feel dread as you walk in, unsure what the day is going to bring. That place that made you realize that bullying didn't stop after you left school. That place where you experience racist or sexist micro-aggressions on a daily basis. That place where they say they are supporting wellbeing and give you a patronizing workshop from a motivational speaker who made you dance to rave music that only served to frustrate you and make you feel worse (yes, talking from experience there).

These are a snapshot of experiences that I have heard about through my work or experienced personally. 'Work' can be many different things to many different people, and creating workplaces that work has been a central part of my recent work (I am a clinical psychologist, don't you know).

The ups and downs of working life

But let's not deride work, because it can be good for your wellbeing and mental health – it can create structure, meaning, financial security, purpose and a sense of achievement.[1] Research shows that working and getting people back to work after a period of illness or leave can have many benefits for their mental health.[2] But work can also be terrible for your mental health and wellbeing, as it can stress you, traumatize you, devalue you, remove your autonomy, make you feel overwhelmed and/or out of control, create impossible demands, leach into other important parts of your life, force you to interact daily with people you would walk away from at a party and, let's face it, can make you feel like utter crap. Work is such a central part of our lives that it has a powerful impact on how we feel and our health (physical and mental). In recent surveys, people said their manager has a bigger impact on their mental health than any other factor[3] and 25 per cent said work has a detrimental impact on their wellbeing.[4] In terms of our burnout tree, the workplace and its culture you step into on a regular basis can be a protective and energizing factor, or it can add so many stressors to your branches that it is inevitable they will start to weigh you down, which can lead to multiple mental and physical health issues and, of course, burnout.

Work, wellbeing and burnout

As we've seen in Chapter 1, traditional paid work has been central to the concept of burnout (although we need to challenge the notion of what work means, and we'll look at that more in the next chapter). There's no getting away from the fact that work, the stress it creates and how this is managed (not just by you but by the organization too), is normally a major contributory factor to burnout.

Work has a critical impact on wellbeing because it's often a large component of our life. It's important to us, it's tied into our purpose, meaning, routine and identity, and, at least for most people, it's a necessity to live. This chapter is mainly about making work work for you. But if you are a leader or manager then it is not just about you, it's about the people who work for you too. Looking after wellbeing in your workplace should be your priority: it's not just good for people (including you), it's also good for business. Workplaces that support wellbeing have reduced staff turnover, better productivity, improved safety outcomes and reduced absenteeism and presenteeism (when we are at work but not really working).[5] It's really a win-win situation.

Research also tells us it impacts on the metrics that matter across a diverse range of industries – including increased profits, better performance on the stock market, improved reputation, attracting better staff, greater creativity and innovation[6] and improved patient outcomes.[7] It's a no-brainer:

looking after wellbeing at work works for everybody. It's impossible to cover here all the factors that contribute to creating a workplace that supports wellbeing (I run a ten-week university course on that and even then, I am skimming the surface), but we will look at some of the key issues that can lead to burnout in the workplace, and ways you can manage them to reduce your (or your employees') risk of burning out.

As you go through this chapter, think about how work-related factors fit into your burnout tree, including the stressors your work creates (the weight in your branches), the workplace context (the weather around your tree) and how your personal factors interact with these workplace stressors to exacerbate or improve them.

WORK AND IDENTITY

I work, therefore I am

'What do you want to be when you grow up?' I can guarantee nearly everyone has been asked or has asked this question. This instills beliefs around work as your main aim, purpose, maybe even ultimate goal. It's no wonder that work is often part of our identity. However, at the extreme we can become defined by our jobs. It can feel like work is not what we do to live, rather it is life and who we are fundamentally. As a child I never said I wanted to be a clinical psychologist when I grew up, but I did say I wanted to be a graphic designer, a teacher, a *National Geographic* photographer (yes, I still want to be that when I grow up), and I knew that my aims were to work, and work hard. I never said I wanted to become any of the things that are really important to me – safe and secure, content, enjoying life, and seeing the world. My answer was always a job I wanted to 'be'. Fast forward to Emma-who-has-grown-up and has somehow not become a photographer but is instead a clinical psychologist.

You will have noticed I said 'I am' a clinical psychologist. Not 'I work as'. Not 'I have trained to be'. I AM. This is risky, because what does it mean when I am no longer able to do the role to the standard I expect? If this is what I am, then it can also become what I am not. And that's exactly what happened. To live up to this identity and be a good worker, I worked long hours, staying late to finish work, taking on extra work and doing everything as best as I could. By doing so, I effectively reinforced my identity as a proud, hard-working clinical psychologist. Ultimately, however, I set myself up to fail, as maintaining my identity in this way was only possible when my life allowed it. When this changed – at first because I had to pick up babies from nursery and then when burnout crash-landed on me – I could no longer keep up this level of energy use or my former (unrealistic) standards. My identity was at risk, and ongoing efforts to maintain it meant I reduced other areas of my life – I really did become just my job. My identity also created barriers to alleviating burnout – it made some sensible solutions seem impossible, like taking leave or just leaving. I WAS my job; therefore, who would I be without it?

You work, therefore you are

You too will likely have answered the same question as me as a child, and for many of you your work will have become integral to your identity as a result. We are successful, as long as we are successful in work. We strive to maintain this identity through effort, time and energy. We stay when we should quit, and we work when we should be building other parts of our identity. Failures in this role become failures of us as a person. It can make us question our identity: if we no longer have this role, then who are we? This loss can take a sledgehammer to our identity. For many of us, our job is synchronized with who we are, and this can make us a fantastic, hardworking and dedicated employee. However, it can also make us a fantastic candidate for burnout, as research tells us that over-identifying with work can put us at risk of burnout.[8]

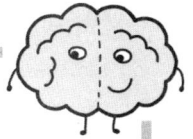

Brian the Brain reflections

- Is your identity enmeshed with your work?
- Has work become all-consuming so that other parts of your identity have been ditched?
- Do you strive to maintain your work identity by working too much/long hours/taking on extra tasks?
- Have any aspects of work created challenges for your identity? This could be leaving work, changing roles, no longer able to work at the level you used to, lack of career progression.
- What other parts of your identity are important?
- How can you build these other parts of your identity?

Work and stress

Let's face it, stress is an inevitable part of work, with its demands, deadlines and pressures. If you work, there will normally be some stressors resulting from your work role in your tree branches (see Chapter 2). This might include deadlines, problems to solve, overwhelm or perhaps boredom, if you feel under-challenged. As always, our personal factors intermingle with these stressors to influence how we cope with them. However, your role and the tasks involved are just one factor that causes stress. It's also important to think about the system and work culture (the weather around your tree) and whether this creates additional stress or exacerbates the inevitable stressors of work and makes you feel worse (more on this shortly).

HOW DO YOU FEEL IN WORK?

Of course, it's not just about stress; we need to think about how work makes us feel generally (I told you emotions were at the heart of everything we do!). This is about both your role and the culture. Do you feel valued, helpfully challenged, supported and safe to raise issues? Or do you feel overworked, at risk, devalued and denigrated? Do you look forward to work or are you filled with the Sunday-night dread of returning to work on Monday? These feelings are indicators of what's going on for you and can help you identify what's working and what's not working.

If you feel great at work, then job done – on to the next chapter. But I suspect you are reading this because you don't, so let's go on a deeper dive.

Brian the Brain reflections

- What stressors does work add to your burnout tree? Think about:
    - Which aspects of your role create stress?
    - Which aspects of the work environment create stress?
    - Does work create stress in any other part of your life (e.g. impact on your home life)?

- How do you manage these stressors?
- In what ways does your workplace help you manage these stressors?
- In what ways does your workplace exacerbate them?
- How do you feel in work? What about when you think about work?
- What contributes to how you feel at and about work?

Workplace systems and burnout

When we think about making work work, it's not just the person that matters, it's the system around them – the physical environment, the processes, the managers, the colleagues and the cultures they create. The culture creates the rules we work by, impacting how we function and feel at work. A toxic culture can pile on stress and weaken our ability to cope, while a supportive culture can help us manage inevitable work stressors and help us cope. Yes, what you do is important, but the context (the weather around your tree) has a critical impact on your burnout tree and, therefore, likelihood of burning out.[9] Focusing solely on individuals and ignoring the context is blameful, unhelpful and ignores causes of burnout. In my workplace wellbeing role, I frequently say that our main aim is not increasing people's ability to cope with detrimental work situations; it is targeting the root cause of what makes them feel this way, and that is the system in which we operate. It is critical for how you work, your health and wellbeing, and for burnout, and we need to address this.

We can't take the person out of the system. Although workplace cultures are critical for burnout, they interact with who we are as a person. The workplace culture can amplify (or mitigate) personal factors that lead to burnout. For example, if you already fear failure or strive for perfectionism, having a critical manager can amplify this, and you may then work harder to feel good enough. If you struggle to ask for support, and when you do your workplace puts the blame back on you, you are likely to not seek support again. These are some of the myriad ways that your individual characteristics and context interact to amplify stress and increase the likelihood of burnout. Recognizing this interaction and taking steps to help you cope is important, but recognizing and thinking about the contextual factors is, I would argue, even more important in our anti-burnout campaign. If we don't, it can lead to gaslighting ourselves, making us feel helpless to tackle issues or using all our energy fighting battles that can't be won. Before I explain this, let's think about some specific workplace factors linked to burnout.

BURNOUT-CREATING SYSTEMS

There's lots of research into workplace factors that support or negatively impact on wellbeing.[10] Factors that enhance wellbeing include:

- Manageable workloads
- Safe and pleasant working environments
- Clear roles, expectations and communication
- Supportive managers or leaders
- Positive relationships with colleagues
- Job security and prospects
- Variety in your role

- Trust and autonomy
- Opportunities to develop
- Minimal work/life interference

None of this should be any surprise – if you've ever been in work, think about what made you feel good and what made you feel stressed or bad. When we look specifically at burnout there are a number of work-related factors for which there's solid research to say they relate to burnout.[11] These are:

- **Workload:** No surprises here. Too much unmanageable work overfills your capacity cup and creates stress. It can also start to impact in other ways: as you use your personal time to catch up, you may stop doing activities you enjoy that mitigate stress. You can feel like you don't have time to do the things in work that support your wellbeing, such as taking breaks, supervision or connecting with colleagues.
- **Value:** Feeling devalued or that work conflicts with your values are risk factors for burnout. At the most extreme, this can become moral injury – trauma resulting from being involved in things that go against your values and ethics.
- **Control:** Feeling a lack of control over what you do can negatively affect your wellbeing at work. Your managers' style matters here: autocratic managers tend to micromanage people, so they feel they have no autonomy over what they do and therefore little control.
- **Reward:** This is, of course, about financial reward – poor pay and job insecurity are major stressors. But it's also about feeling rewarded in your role, because you feel you are doing a good job and are appreciated for your work. Perceiving an imbalance between the effort you put in and the reward you receive, especially if you are highly committed to your job, increases your risk of burnout.

- **Community:** This is about the people around you at work. Do you feel part of a supportive team and are you able to share issues and ask for support? If not, a lack of a supportive community can contribute to burnout.
- **Fairness:** Unfair treatment causes resentment, discomfort between colleagues and upset. A colleague being paid more for doing the same job will piss you off, as will someone being promoted who everyone knows is no good at their job. But there's also the more sinister stuff, such as being treated unfairly because of your sex, race or mental health. Then there's bullying and harassment, which are inherently unfair, stressful and often psychologically damaging. Unfairness results in stress and makes us distrust our workplace and feel devalued.

THE GENERAL CULTURE

The work culture sets the tone for how we operate in the workplace and can be a major risk factor for burnout. Many of the factors that contribute to burnout often occur as a result of poor culture. We can think of cultures on a continuum from psychologically safe (that support wellbeing) to toxic blame cultures that are detrimental to wellbeing.[12]

Psychological safety is a concept coined by scholar Amy Edmondson which is 'the belief that you won't be ousted or humiliated when you speak up with ideas, concerns or mistakes'.[13] A psychologically safe culture is one in which you feel safe, trusted, respected and comfortable asking questions, speaking up and seeking support. Not surprisingly, this is linked to improved individual and team performance and wellbeing.[14] This concept demonstrates the link between how we feel at work and how we operate, including how we tackle issues and manage stressors. This is important, because operating in a psychologically safe culture reduces risk of burnout.[15]

The opposite of this is a blame (or toxic) culture. In these cultures, we feel unsupported, not respected, and fearful of speaking up as we will be criticized and blamed as fault is apportioned for mistakes and errors. This results in us being reluctant to raise issues, take risks, speak out or accept responsibility for our actions, because we are afraid of what might happen. Toxic work cultures can also be characterized by other factors such as bullying, harassment, unprofessional behaviours, micromanagement, autocratic leadership styles, poor communication, unrealistic expectations, negativity and lack of support. Research demonstrates that these types of cultures are linked to unnecessary stress, physical and mental health issues[16] and, of course, burnout.[17]

But what if the culture and system is me?

When we think about work, a traditional workplace often comes to mind, but that's just not the reality for many of us. You might work remotely, be freelance or self-employed – and each of these scenarios creates different challenges and stressors. The risk factors for burnout may also vary, such as juggling multiple roles, greater crossover of work and home life, lack of financial or job security and/or lack of colleagues for support. However, being in at least some of these roles can also provide opportunities. It's not that burnout is less likely to happen, but you can have more influence and power to create the system and culture that you want. You do not have to take ideas to a manager for approval and there are no layers of bureaucracy to navigate to implement a change. I'm not saying change is easy, as there will still be multiple barriers to shifting your own personal work culture. But if it's not working for you, you often have the autonomy and power to shift it.

However, recognizing this can also come with a big slice of shame (like I experienced), because if you ARE the system, you can believe you are very much to blame for your burnout, as it was caused by the system you created. Let's diminish the shame – we all get into patterns and behaviours that don't work for us for many different reasons (I wouldn't have a job if we didn't). Don't waste your energy on shame. Instead, use your energy and opportunity to create a system that works for you.

> **Anti-burnout Exercise 12:**
> **Observing the work weather around your burnout tree**
>
> Look at the factors that contribute to wellbeing and burnout and think if any of these apply to your workplace:
>
> - How would you describe the culture at your work (the weather in the clouds)?
> - Now think about which factors in your workplace environment negatively impact on you and increase your risk of burnout (the lightning).
> - Which factors at work positively contribute to your wellbeing and are protective against burnout (the sun)?
> - Now think about how these factors impact on you: How do they make you feel? How do they impact on your behaviour? Do they impact on your life, including out-of-work hours?

Making work work for you

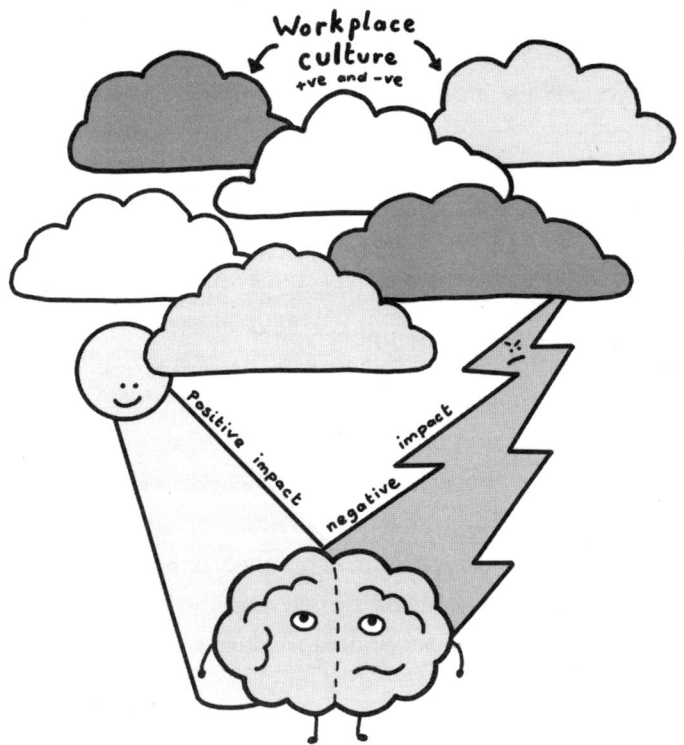

IMPACT OF A TOXIC CULTURE

Now let's think of some ways toxic cultures fuel burnout. This one is obvious: they load your branches with stressors, creating chronic stress and a range of not very nice emotions that, over time, weaken or crush your tree. They might also amplify or create beliefs that are unhelpful and lead to behaviours that inadvertently make you feel worse. However, let's look at some of the more insidious and specific ways they can fuel burnout.

Feeling helpless and learned helplessness

One of the factors that can lead to burnout is a lack of control and feeling helpless to create change. This can happen for many reasons: because the culture makes it hard to raise issues, because you've tried and it's had minimal or no impact, or you are unsure the effort is worth the outcome. As a result you feel despondent, trapped and powerless to change things. Ultimately this can lead to learned helplessness: when you do not believe your actions can change a situation and give up trying, because what's the point (even though there may be things you can do)? Learned helplessness really isn't good for people, and can contribute to burnout.[18]

When I read about learned helplessness, I often think its portrayed as some sort of personal characteristic. However, this is normally an adaptive response to a situation, as keeping on trying to make things change with little impact is stressful and exhausting. I can say this from personal experience, because this is part of what lay the groundwork for my burnout. Normally I will not stand for poor workplace behaviour and like to tackle problems head on and change things for the better. But this takes time, effort and energy, often above and beyond your normal work role. If nothing changes as a result, things get worse or the outcome is blatantly unfair (e.g. promotion for someone whose behavior is unacceptable), you have to question whether the time, stress and energy use are worth it in a situation where you have to stay, and therefore survive, for the time being at least.

I had a few specific experiences that made me feel helpless, but can you imagine how people feel if they experience constant belittling, bullying, discrimination, racism or harassment? This is stressful in itself but becomes even more problematic in a situation where you feel you cannot influence change and have little choice but to stay in that environment for whatever reason – financial being the most common. Wellbeing books can say 'you have a choice'. I often think this reflects a privileged point of view that fails to recognize not everyone has the same choices. We can't all take a break from work and we don't all have the option to change jobs. Now, don't feel ashamed if you are able to change your work environment – that's amazing! But for many people these traps are not just in their minds: they have limited choices because of financial or practical constraints. So, let's not pathologize finding it hard to change or think of learned helplessness as some sort of failure; sometimes it is hard. The exercise on page 138 looks at both determining what you can change and how you can cope with those aspects you can't change immediately.

Gaslighting yourself: Internalizing a negative culture as something wrong with you

Toxic cultures are insidious and can be hard to make sense of. Rarely is someone going to stand up and say, 'This is the culture round here.' Cultures hide in what people do and say, to create the collective beliefs about how we should behave. The sneaky nature of cultures means it's hard to point the finger at them. Instead, we can gaslight ourselves: we blame the failures to fit in, keep up or cope on ourselves rather than the system.

Turning on ourselves and believing it is something about us is called 'internal causal attribution' and it is, sadly, a classic outcome when people have been bullied[19] – they internalize it to be something inherently wrong with them. However, toxic and poor cultures also have this effect. In these cultures, when things go wrong the individual is blamed, either directly or indirectly (this is the reason they are often called 'blame cultures'). I've seen this happen many times: perhaps a member of staff raises their excessively high, unmanageable workload and they are told they need to develop better time-management skills. Rather than recognizing where the issue actually lies and what the manager or organization can do by way of support, the person is told this is their problem and they need to do better. This can be thought of as a form of organizational gaslighting: if you make the person believe it's their problem, you absolve organizational or managerial responsibility to change. It is no surprise that people start to gaslight and blame themselves. Instead of correctly pinpointing the external issue, it instead becomes something about us, an inherent failure or something we need to learn to manage. It's common to do this, and usually we don't even realize we are doing it.

We are more at risk of turning on ourselves if we are already highly critical of and blame ourselves when things go wrong, are sensitive to failure or don't have supportive relationships that help us gain another perspective. Poor cultures have a knack of doing this: the responsibility to change and the blame for failing is placed on the person.

The exercise on page 138 is designed to help with learned helplessness and gaslighting ourselves by correctly pinpointing the issues and identifying what is within our power to change.

Taking action to make work work

Let's spend some time thinking about how we can make work work for you. This is a mini formulation to make sense of work and pinpoint what you can do. To do this we are going to mainly think about the weather around your tree (the systemic and cultural factors), break them down a bit more and categorize them by identifying:

- Personal factors within your control, such as your behaviours.
- Systemic factors that you could influence or take action on – we can break these down further into:
  - Hares: things that can be targeted quickly to effect change.
  - Tortoises: things that may take more time, or which you can only influence gradually or slightly.
- Systemic factors that you see no way to shift.

Recognizing the systemic issues and categorizing them in this way helps us understand the situation and clearly see where we can use our energy beneficially to effect change. This can make us feel better in a number of ways. It helps us understand the issues and see what we can do about them, which makes us feel more in control. It clearly pinpoints where the issues are, which stops us from blaming ourselves for things that aren't our fault or thinking we are fundamentally flawed and need to do better. It stops us wasting energy battling unwinnable wars and frees our minds and energy to take action where it matters, which can reduce helplessness and increase hope. Finally, when things are out of our control, it enables us to find ways to cope (if we have to) or consider moving ourselves to different weather.

You will notice I have not predominately focused on individual ways you can get better at managing your work, such as time management or productivity hacks. This is intentional, because focusing efforts to change the individual in an unhelpful context propagates the myth that it is your responsibility to do better and cope, instead of recognizing the systemic factors. We should not put the responsibility on individuals to endure, persevere and be resilient in toxic, dysfunctional and broken structures and systems. It's the system that needs to change.

There may of course be things you could do differently, and you may find techniques around increasing resilience, productivity and improving how you work helpful (I've included some great Further Reading on page 306 if you want to do this). By all means, think about these under the category 'what I can control', but also ensure you are not using this as a stick with which to blame and beat yourself up.

Anti-burnout Exercise 13: Correctly locating where the issues exist

You have already thought about stressors, the system and culture at work. Now use the image opposite to break this down a bit more into the following categories:

1. Personal factors within your control.
2. Systemic factors that you could take action around (hares and tortoises).
3. Systemic factors that you see no way to shift.

Now you have divided this up, let's look at some ideas for things you can do to help in each category. You will also have your own ideas, so add them to the list too.

1. Personal factors within your control

- **Build your identity outside work** – Do things that shift your focus from work, that you enjoy and that build your identity.
- **Take time to regularly reflect** – What have you done well? What is causing you stress? What can you do about this?

Making work work for you

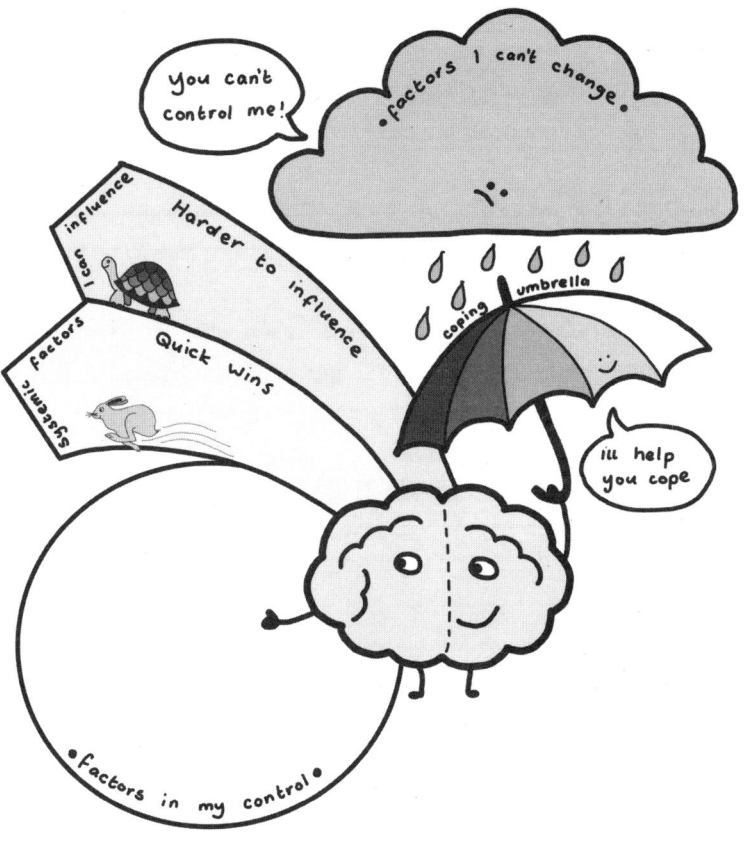

- **Switching off** – Make sure you find ways to switch from work brain to a more relaxed state: a ritual that marks the end of the day and signals to your brain you are now switching off. If you work from home this might mean tidying away your work area from sight.
- **Manage work/life interference** – Find ways to ensure non-work time isn't encroached on by work. Set 'out of offices'. Mute work WhatsApp groups. Remove email access from your phone. Have a separate work and personal telephone.

- **End the day with clarity** - Focus on what you have achieved and have a clear focus of what you need to do next.
- **Don't buy into cultural edicts** - Does everyone leave late or not take breaks? This is the culture playing out through behaviour. Set your own culture! Just take the goddam break, leave on time and see what happens. We have a lot to learn from Danish culture as a model of how to work and there are some great reads in the reading list on page 306.
- For goodness' sake, **TAKE THE BREAK** - Breaks during the day, lunch breaks, holidays, parental leave, carer's leave. Take them all. This is one of the strongest factors that supports employee wellbeing and reduces burnout. The system won't fail with you not there, and if it does, it highlights an issue in the system that needs to be addressed, which you have been masking by not taking breaks.
- **What energizes you at work** - Can you build more on this? And reduce more of the things that deplete you?

2. Changing the system

(Be aware you need to think about your energy levels and time because doing this can contribute to burnout, and it's a balance.) Remember to divide these issues and corresponding solutions into quick wins (hares) and tortoises (take longer/harder to influence). Starting with quick wins can motivate you to take on the more gradual stuff.

- **Recognize what you can't change** - Conserve your energy from fighting the useless fight.

Making work work for you

- **Control the things you can control** – Do what is within your control to help you deal with the situation. This might be declining unnecessary meetings or having prepared ways to respond to certain behaviours in meetings. It might be identifying a mentor or just making sure you look after yourself well by eating, hydrating, switching off and resting.
- **Develop community** – Find your like-minded souls who give you support and with whom you can talk things through. Set up supportive groups – an informal lunch group, a more formal supervision group or a group focusing on specific issues, such a neurodiversity or menopause, that gives people a louder voice to raise issues.
- **Raise things** – Don't assume that just because you've noticed an issue, other people will too. Raise it in a meeting. Send an email about it. Find the right person to discuss it with.
- **Suggest solutions** – What do people need to work well? Can you create this change, or can you suggest that this change be created?
- **Know and access your supports** – What systems are in place to share employee voices? Are there feedback mechanisms or specific meetings? Are there places or people in the system to support you with this?

3. Raise your umbrellas: systemic factors that you can't shift

For these, you need to think how you can protect yourself using your umbrella to reduce impact and help you cope.

- **Depersonalize work** – Find ways to switch off work,

reduce overidentification with it and increase your identity elsewhere. Notice self-blame - use this exercise to correctly locate the problem where it exists. Talk things through with a supportive person who can help look at the situation in different ways.

- **Know your rights and supports** - Be clear on what your rights are and when something has transgressed them. Know the mechanisms for raising unacceptable behaviour, such as complaints or employee voice procedures, and who can help, such as trade unions or employee groups/networks.
- **Talk things through** - The more you hide things, the more you are likely to blame and shame yourself. Talk through how you feel with someone you trust. This may be a professional or a friend. Many occupations have access to independent external supports that can help you in talking through issues and/or how you feel.
- **Consider change** - Think about the barriers to change and what's stopping you. Often change can feel risky; the status quo can seem the better, safer option, when it actually it might not be. It can be helpful to think this through with other people and explore other options.
- **Know when to leave. Have a plan** - You need to weigh up when a job is having a more detrimental than beneficial impact on you. Your health is valuable and can't always be changed once it goes wrong. Plan what the next steps are for when you come to this decision and, if you can, put things in place to help you make it (such as some savings, contacting job agencies and planning how you will cope with your family).

Anti-burnout takeaways

- Work can have a significant impact on your health and wellbeing, and work-related stress can put you at risk of burnout.
- The culture you work in and how it makes you feel is the most significant factor contributing to burnout.
- Workplace risk factors for burnout include: workload, level of control, whether you feel valued and rewarded, fairness and the community you have around you.
- Over-identifying with work can be a factor that makes you more likely to work in ways that contribute to burnout.
- The workplace system can lead to you feeling helpless or blaming yourself for external factors, which can contribute to burnout.
- Recognizing the workplace factors that are contributing to your stress is critical to understand which type of actions to take to support you.
- The action you take to make work work will depend on whether these factors are personal factors, systemic factors you can change or systemic factors that are unlikely to change.

Chapter 7
Who cares? Caring and the other roles in our lives

What do you care about? What comes to mind in response to this question? Most commonly, it will be other meaningful people in our lives, and most of us will play a caring role throughout our lives, whether that be through work or personal connections. We may care for sick people, children and other family members. We may also care about meaningful activities to us, the wider world or social justice issues.

Don't switch off at this point if you are not a traditional carer, such as a parent or nurse, because we nearly all care in one way or another, or will do at one point in our lives. Human brains are designed for us to be social, and caring is essential for relationships: it creates bonds, helps us thrive and makes societies work. Caring can be wonderful, meaningful and positive, but it can also be stressful, exhausting, overwhelming, undervalued, unrecognized and demanding.

Care can add to the stressors in your burnout tree and deplete your energy and body budget with very little time to top it up, increasing risk of burnout. In whichever way you care, it's important to recognize the impact of it, so we can become anti-burnout in these essential roles.

A day in the life of the motherhood juggle

My children are slightly older now, so this is easier than it used to be, but I'm sure my typical day a few years ago will sound familiar to any parent. I'd start by super-speedily getting myself ready (I got it down to four minutes at one point), as well as getting children ready who refused to put certain socks on and didn't worry about suppressing their emotional reaction when you gave them the wrong colour plate. Then I wrangled drop-offs, found a parking space at a busy hospital (nearly impossible), before starting my clinic at 9am. I felt like I had worked a whole day before I even started work – doing this without bursting into tears was a huge success. Having to sit down and crush that morning's frazzled feeling to take in the traumatic stories I was hearing was quite the cognitive effort.

But this was just the start. I had to get through the day on the back of disrupted sleep (sometimes less than three hours, as sleeping wasn't a key skill on my children's CVs) and ensure I did the job I cared a lot about – caring for a lot for people – at the standard that met my values. There was often very little time for breaks, in a demanding job, with little fuel (I reckon I was constantly chronically dehydrated) and I never finished my 'to do' list by the end of the day.

Then the evening work started: nursery pick-up, cooking, negotiating meal times with children, managing their emotions after exhausting days, singing songs to coax them into the bath, cuddling them and watching *In the Night Garden* (this was the best bit), then bedtime books (which I also loved), then getting children who didn't like to sleep to sleep, then attempting to bring a modicum of control to the chaos of home and prepare for the next day. Then switching off. Nah, not really, just falling into a slump of exhaustion and then finally getting to bed to be only ever partly asleep, as I was on constant alert throughout the night. Then parental Groundhog Day: a few short hours of disrupted sleep later, get up to start it all over again.

At the time, I don't even think I realized how hard this was (as is the case for most mothers). The tantalizing mythical THERE was omnipresent – if only I could master the right sleep technique, meal prep, bedtime routine, parenting hack, time management technique, then I would master this parenting malarky, get life in balance and feel in control again. I saw it as something I could overcome and achieve, if only I tried harder and was good enough – but of course, this was an unrealistic goal, and ultimately it just wasted more energy that I didn't have.

I wonder now, looking back, if I was burned out then. I lived in a fugue for several years: my brain was permanently exhausted yet alert to respond to my children, and my cognition was malfunctioning (lack of sleep will do that to you), meaning simple tasks were often difficult. I want to cuddle the past me and tell her how well she is doing. She was finding it difficult not because she was doing anything wrong or needed to do better, but just because it was hard.

PARENTAL BURNOUT

We need to recognize that parenting is cognitively, emotionally and often physically demanding – and its tasks and responsibilities could rightfully be considered 'work'. However, often this work is unrecognized, undervalued and poorly supported by societal structures, which can make for an even more difficult experience. Caring for children with additional needs or medical conditions is an even more demanding task.

Being a parent is equally rewarding and challenging, as we navigate the ups and downs and constantly evolving demands, from a tiny crying bundle through tantrumming toddler to Taylor Swift-obsessed preteen, tech-obsessed teen, then young adults leaving home (or perhaps still with us). I would say parenting is like the longest game of Snakes and Ladders in the world. You are perpetually guessing how to respond to an ever-changing landscape, throwing the dice, hoping that you will get the next move right. The square you land on can bring a random mix of love, joy and pride, but it might also bring you worry, stress and guilt, or an epic tantrum in response to a tiny imperceivable mistake (it was a bad move to make those baked beans touch the fish fingers). Just as we feel we've mastered one route, the route changes, with a new developmental twist or a surprise parenting challenge, and we slide down a ladder to feel like a complete novice again, back at square one. And we do all this with our capacity cup (see Chapter 3) always nearly full, so that even the tiniest extra unexpected addition thrown into our cup can make it overflow.

With perpetual challenges and demands to juggle, we rarely get a chance to switch off, our body budget is often depleted and our burnout tree is frequently groaning under the weight of its branches. Given this, it's no surprise that parents are more likely to experience burnout. Mothers, single parents, parents of ill, disabled or neurodivergent children, and those without family or childcare support are even more likely to burn out.[1] It's such a common experience that research has started to look at whether we should consider parental burnout a phenomenon in itself.[2]

Although these parental zombies display similar characteristics as the burnout zombies we've already met, they may have some specific characteristics that are unique to them. Their symptoms can relate to parental responsibilities, for example they may no longer enjoy being with their child and disengage emotionally from them.[3] Parental burnout can also result in a difficult dose of feelings about yourself as a parent or your children. Research tells us we should take parental burnout very seriously, because it can have significant health or mental health consequences.[4]

OTHER UNPAID CARE ROLES

Of course, it's not just caring for children that can create an imbalance between resources and demands to overflow our capacity cup. Throughout my career, I have worked with unpaid carers, often family members, and have seen the immense impact this role can have. This might be caring for elderly parents, a partner who has an illness or injury, or supporting friends. Over half (57 per cent) of unpaid carers report feeling overwhelmed most of the time.[5] There are never-ending 'to do' lists and constant cognitive demands: anticipating, planning and organizing; learning new skills; working out what to do. There are the emotional demands, the worry, supporting difficult emotions in others; navigating complex care or health systems; constant appointments; not getting the support you need; and the financial impact.[6] Then there are the physical demands and impact: the exhaustion, low mood, lack of sleep. All these demands put carers at greater risk of burnout and other health conditions.[7]

Finally, there's the lack of time or support for your own needs, which often come at the bottom of the pile. While unpaid care keeps societies functioning, often it's not recognized in practices, policies and support services. I've worked with many unpaid carers, and they have told me they feel overlooked, and the lack of support means there are fewer levers to alleviate the pressure.

CARING AS A PROFESSION

Let's be honest, most people don't go into a caring profession because they are driven by money; most are driven by values and helping people, because these jobs are often underpaid, highly demanding and stressful. From working in health and social care for many years, I know it's filled with predominantly highly empathetic people who enter this profession because it meets their values – they truly care and want to make a difference. But I also see a group of people who are at high risk of burnout[8] because of the very fact that they *care*.

Working in care is a high-demand role for our brain and body – not only are these jobs often physically demanding but they are also emotionally exhausting and can take their toll. You are dealing with emotionally demanding situations, difficult emotions (in yourself and others) and emotionally complex tasks, such as communicating difficult news. Often people will work long hours to ensure they can deliver care at the standard they want to, increasing work/life interference. Trauma can be a normal part of the role: you can witness or hear about more trauma in one month, or even one day, than most people would in a lifetime. However, you are also susceptible to being worn out because you cannot care in the way you want to, due to systemic pressures or the overwhelming demands in the role. This creates a stressful values conflict, which at its worst can lead to moral injury, a traumatic response stemming from a perceived moral transgression on the part of yourself or others. We know from the research that moral injury increased in health and care workers during the pandemic as they were unable to deliver care at their desired standard.[9]

So, we've got a mix of people who really care about helping, paired with a job that often makes impossible demands to help, with insufficient resources. Surprise, surprise – care workers are more at risk of burnout than the general working population.[10]

SUPER HELPERS

Research highlights that there can be personal factors that intrinsically make some people very dedicated carers, but this may be detrimental to them long term. While it's not a clinical diagnosis, the term 'super helper' (sometimes called 'rescuer syndrome') is used to recognize a set of characteristics.

'Super helper syndrome' is a term coined by Baker and Vincent[11] to describe someone who feels compelled to help others to the detriment of their own needs, and whose identity and worth are tied into supporting others. This is driven by the belief that you must help others and suppress your own needs, to be a good person. If you are a 'super helper', you may have very high standards and feel guilty that you are never doing enough. You spend a lot of energy and time on helping people and feel compelled to help or offer help, yet accept and receive very little help yourself. This can be exhausting and lead to being taken advantage of (or even exploitation) and self-criticism. Constantly helping others while negating your own needs can gradually wear down your burnout tree – there are too many demands and you are not building enough strength to manage them.

Who cares?

CARING FOR YOURSELF WITH ILLNESS OR A DISABILITY

An often overlooked part of the caring conversation is the demands of looking after yourself, particularly when you have a chronic condition, illness or disability. Many of us are not very good at caring for ourselves, but when we have additional health or support needs, it is even more necessary to do so, even though it may be more challenging and demanding.

A condition in itself can have a physical, emotional and often cognitive impact (fatigue is extremely common with many conditions), which can mean less energy and time, effectively shrinking your capacity cup. Additional demands related to managing the condition can deplete you further and may include: stress and worry, advocating for yourself, having to plan constantly to manage the condition, frequent medical appointments, treatment regimes, circumnavigating a world not designed for your needs and navigating complex health and social care systems. This results in a scenario where you have to manage greater demands, often with reduced capacity. In addition, limited time and energy means other protective factors that help you cope often fall to the wayside, such as social networks and hobbies, thereby increasing stress further.

CARING FOR THE WORLD

There's a lot to care about in the world right now, from climate crisis to racism, discrimination, poverty, wars and famines. Experiencing these directly is, of course, a major stressor that can impact our burnout tree, but caring from afar can have an impact too. We should care about these things even if they don't influence us directly, but this can have an emotional cost. The nature of our technological world means it's difficult to switch off from crises, and constantly feeling empathy for the distress of billions of people in the world is overwhelming and exhausting. Remember, too, that stress feels worse when it seems unrelenting, unmanageable and out of control – and that's certainly the case when disasters stream at us perpetually through non-stop media. This can make us question our values and beliefs or even question humanity, leaving us feeling hopeless and helpless, like there is no good in the world and nothing we can do about it, all of which can take an emotional toll.

The cost of empathy – compassion fatigue

Giving care can be beneficial to us – it can build social networks, support wellbeing and has helped humans throughout history. However, it can also deplete us. This can be particularly true if we have high levels of empathy, when we can see the world through other people's eyes and feel what they feel. Among our burned-out zombies, we have a group who were previously incredibly compassionate and deeply invested in caring. This has exhausted them to the point they no longer have the same levels of compassion, empathy or ability to care – known as 'compassion fatigue'. It is a particular risk for healthcare professionals and those in caring roles, and it is tied to their strong values in helping others. These zombies may have been the previous super-helper, or just caring people whose values and identity are intrinsically tied into caring.

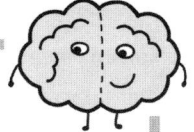

> **Brian the Brain reflections:**
> **What cost does caring have on you?**
>
> - What caring roles do you have? (Think about caring for others and for yourself, particularly if you have a chronic condition.)
> - What support do you have around you to help you care?
> - In what ways does caring create deposits in your body budget?
> - In what ways does caring create withdrawals from your body budget?
> - Do your caring responsibilities impact on your ability to care for your own needs?
> - Is your capacity cup constantly almost full or overflowing due to caring responsibilities?
> - Do you feel high levels of empathy? How does this impact on you?
> - Do you recognize any of the aspects of super-helper syndrome in yourself?
> - How do these aspects of caring feed into your burnout tree formulation?

The mental load and burnout

Hold on, I have to take a call from school now before we go on to the next section. Yes, of course, school always calls me first, and it's usually my work that is impacted as a result. While we absolutely need to recognize the impact of caring on all people, we also need to address that caring roles are still disproportionately carried out by women.[12]

Caring roles are part of the domestic load, which we know still falls predominantly to women.[13] Time and again, research shows that women are more likely to burn out, and one reason for this is thought to be the disproportionate distribution of the domestic and mental load.

WHAT IS THE MENTAL LOAD?

My mum worked while I was growing up. I remember at one point, with three children, she was doing a law degree, working in the university library in the evenings, and doing the majority of the care work. I was proud of her; she was a strong woman making her own choices and was (and still is) my role model. It's only now that I imagine her mental load and how exhausted she must have been (but I guess as it was Scotland in the 1980s and 1990s, nobody really spoke about this).

My mum was doing much more than going to work and university and looking after us. She was planning and anticipating, thinking how and when we would get home from school, what we would have for dinner, whether she needed to buy anything for this and prepare it for when she went to work. Such things would have been on her mind from early morning to late at night. But it wasn't just practical stuff; she was the one who anticipated and responded to our emotional needs, talked with us when big emotions came up, took phone calls from clueless teenagers, guided us through problems, picked us up when things went wrong, found lost concert tickets and generally found solutions. She was the invisible planner, anticipator, problem solver and emotion tender that made things work. Like most other women my age I know, I appear to have modelled this and continue to hold the majority of the invisible reigns that keep things ticking along smoothly.

Keeping a household running can be thought to require two distinct but interrelated kinds of labour: the domestic and the mental.[14] Domestic labour is the execution of a task (i.e. dropping children off at school). Mental load refers to the invisible elements of keeping a household functioning – the anticipating, planning and problem-solving required for the tasks to occur. If we break this down a bit more, we can think of two factors to the mental load.

Cognitive load: The planning, anticipating and thinking about all the practical elements of household responsibilities, including organizing playdates, shopping and planning activities. For example, for my mum that would have been planning and preparing the meals for when she was at work.

Emotional load: This includes maintaining the family's emotions, worrying about things, calming things down or just generally tending to the emotional needs of children and other family members. In my story at the start of this chapter, this might be planning activities to keep kids calm on the way home from nursery, distracting them to get them into the bath, or even thinking about their needs when at work. There's also some research to show that women suppress their emotions and needs more than men to make family life work[15] (and we know that suppressing emotions creates greater stress).

Women tend to do more of the domestic load, but the discrepancy is even greater for the mental load,[16] the more invisible elements such as anticipation, planning and research. This really stands out when I speak to my female friends and colleagues – we normally anticipate and plan for family needs such as meals, school snacks, trips and holidays. One doctor friend of mine told me about the time she came home exhausted after a long day at the hospital seeing patients when her husband wasn't working. As she stepped through the door, her husband asked her what was for tea and she exploded and then felt guilty and even more stressed (because women aren't supposed to get angry).

The mental load is invisible, difficult to quantify, boundaryless and unlimited.[17] This means it is like a never-ending tap pouring into your capacity cup (which is, of course, limited). We can't contain it and it spills into every aspect of our lives, and there is no clocking off or a finish point where you can turn off the tap. Considering it this way shows why our capacity cups are constantly overwhelmed, and we often don't even get or give ourselves credit as the work is invisible and difficult to quantity. As I would now say to my younger self: it's not your fault you feel overwhelmed, it is overwhelming.

Just as the mental load is endless, I have endless stories about how the mental load plays out in women's lives. Many things have contributed to this, including traditional gender roles and beliefs, as well as the lack of societal value and recognition of this invisible glue, which not only keeps families going but keeps society going too.

We really need the domestic and mental load to be more evenly split to truly become an anti-burnout world. Research shows that in heterosexual couples, women still take on the majority of the domestic and mental load in a household,[18] while in LGBTQ couples, the load is more evenly distributed.[19] While this varies across cultures, in the UK the Office of National Statistics found that women shoulder 60 per cent more unpaid work annually than men.[20] Similar stats emerge across different countries, which all point to the unpaid, unseen and unrecognized work predominately falling to women, even if they are doing as much paid work.

Who cares?

Anti-burnout Exercise 14: The domestic- and mental-load iceberg

- Think about what the domestic load looks like in your house: these are all the tasks above the water.
- Now think about the invisible mental load required to do these tasks: these are the tasks below the water. If you are struggling to identify them (it can be hard!), there are a number of resources that can help you in the Further Reading on page 306.
- If you want to take this one step further, think of how things are divided up in your household – who is responsible for what?

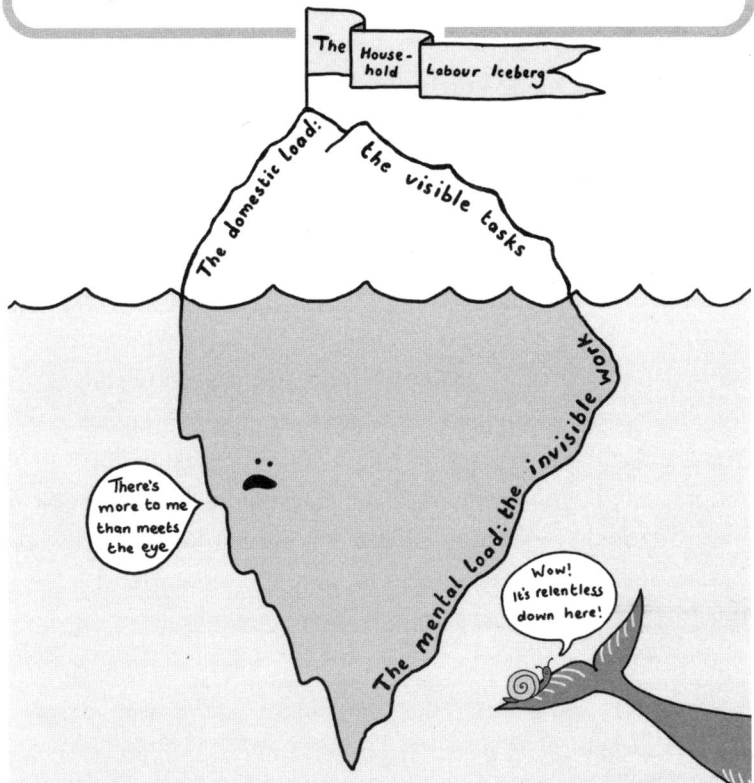

The impact of the mental load

Why is the mental load important when we consider burnout? Research indicates that mothers are more stressed, tired and less happy than fathers.[21] This means at a critical period of their children's development, mothers are often feeling an overwhelming burden. And this burden does discriminate, because for those who have less resources to reduce or manage it, such as monetary resources or access to familial or other social support network, it is an even greater burden.[22]

And it's not just mothers, or even women, who are impacted – for many people, managing the unlimited load is stressful. If there is too much load for too long in our branches, and we cannot turn off the tap to stop more coming in, then it is overwhelming and our branches will eventually break. Furthermore, if we don't recognize the mental load, then we can think there is something fundamentally wrong with us (and Shane rears his nasty head), rather than recognizing the atmospheric pressure constantly mounting around our tree.

How to tackle the mental load?

Well, that's a big question! The very start is to recognize the mental load so that we stop blaming and shaming ourselves for what are structural and societal issues impacting on us. There are some great resources out there for tackling the mental load in your personal life, including the *Fair Play* book and card deck* (and there are more in Further Reading on page 306). However, whenever tackling the mental load is raised, I fear we are just setting women another task to be

---

* A card deck with aspects of the mental load on each card so you can go through them, working out who does what and dividing them up more equally.

responsible for, thereby just adding to their mental load with a difficult, or impossible, task. In fact, the responsibility here is much wider than women's – we all need to take action. As a society we need to value unpaid work and address the mental load. That is not just as individuals – while we can take action to address this in our own spaces, we also need to address this through our societal structures and policies.[23] We need to raise generations who view things differently: we can't just tell girls they can have it all; we need to raise boys who will take on some of the mental load without having to be asked. But I fear we will be waiting a long time for this structural change to happen, so let's first stop and reflect, but also think what we can do as individuals in the here and now.

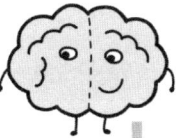

Brian the Brain reflections

- How does the mental load impact on you? What about other family members?
- How does the mental load impact on your relationship?
- What have you tried to manage the mental load? What do you/other people need to do to make this happen?
- Are there ways you can reduce the mental load even just a little? Can you outsource anything? Can you ask for help with anything?
- Do you internalize the mental load by blaming yourself for not managing when actually the load is impossible to manage?
- Can you shift your expectations about yourself?

The systems around our caring roles and burnout

Let's turn back to the system in which our burnout tree operates. I came across a quote by Dr Pooja Lakshmin (in her book *Real Self Care*[24]) while researching for this book:

I hypothesized that what we had all been calling burnout was actually something different – it was societal betrayal ... While burnout places the blame (and thus the responsibility) on the individual and tells women they aren't resilient enough, betrayal points directly to the broken structures around them.

You will remember when we looked at work in the last chapter, we very much focused on the systems in which you operate, because research indicates these are main contributory factors to burnout. The same can be applied to caring work: the system and whether this supports us or undermines us is critical for how we cope. We know that systems which support parents and carers lead to better mental health (and more productive societies, but that's for another book).[25] In contrast to this, the individualistic push in society tells us we should take personal responsibility to do better and become more resilient to cope. This flawed narrative makes us believe we are responsible for how we are feeling, and that we need to do better or take on more to manage this, ironically increasing our load and making us feel worse rather than better. Therefore, me giving you individualistic strategies to manage time better, or do better in some way, would just play into this flawed narrative. There are always things we can change or tweak as individuals, but we need to recognize the weather around our tree (the system), as this creates the conditions that critically put us at risk of burnout.

WHAT CAN WE DO, REALISTICALLY?

Recognizing how the wider systems around us contribute to our burnout is helpful, because it turns an internal ME problem into a wider society issue. This can help lift the weight of self-blame and locate the problems where they really exist. In her brilliant book *All in Her Head*, Misty Pratt says:

It was never about us and our personal failures, maybe burnout is a reasonable reaction to overwhelming demands?[26]

However, acknowledging this can also be hard: it may make you feel out of control or helpless to change – it's difficult to take action and change a larger system (especially when you are perpetually exhausted and barely have energy for day-to-day tasks). So how can we manage the reality of the situations in which we exist in a meaningful way that feels possible and doesn't create additional unrealistic demands? The following exercises are not the answer, but they are all designed with this dilemma in mind.

Anti-burnout Exercise 15: Tiny boosts to your capacity

Look, if you have time, resources and the support to go to a spa (and you enjoy it; I hate spas), then great. But realistically, most carers have very little time to do something big that makes them feel good. Instead, we need to take tiny moments to increase our capacity. This is taking intentional moments during the day to do things that make us feel good, in the knowledge that even tiny boosts can help us get through the day. Each single boost doesn't feel like much, but it can give you a bit more capacity, or make you feel slightly better, to help you get through the next moment, and over time these build up to have a bigger impact on your capacity and wellbeing.

Use the table to think about which tiny boosts you might include and when you could do them. You might need to shift behaviours and challenge beliefs in order to do so (see Chapter 4), and prioritize them over other activities, such as tidying up when your baby sleeps. But we must prioritize them, because the tiny boosts help us deal with what we need to deal with, and make our burnout tree stronger.

A tiny boost that would help me

....

....

When can I do this?

....

....

Who cares?

What are the barriers to doing this?

....

....

How can I make this happen?

....

....

Anti-burnout Exercise 16:
The 'tiny thing' tsunami

This is a tale of a teeny-tiny cute innocent thing and your capacity cup. It is a cautionary tale for when you feel compelled to take on just one more tiny thing that doesn't seem like a big deal: it's just tiny, it will take only five minutes.

Don't be deceived by this tiny thing's innocence. Yes, if you have capacity this tiny thing has minimal impact, but if you are already full (like most carers are) then it poses a critical risk. This tiny thing can result in your capacity cup overflowing in a tsunami wave into overwhelm land, where you are drowning in demands and unable to stay afloat. This cautionary tale is designed to make you stop and think about that teeny-tiny thing that seems so innocent but could have meteoric consequences.

This exercise is about inhibiting your default yes and instead considering if you really have space for the tiny thing and the impact of saying yes. It's about stopping guilt in its tracks and thinking not only about what you should do but also about the potential impact. The research shows that women particularly feel guilty about not taking on extra roles and frequently take on voluntary roles despite it being detrimental to them (school parents committee, anyone?). Store this in your head and use this 'teeny-tiny thing' exercise when you next notice the urge to add something to your cup, and instead of automatically adding it or doing the thing, STOP and really think it through.

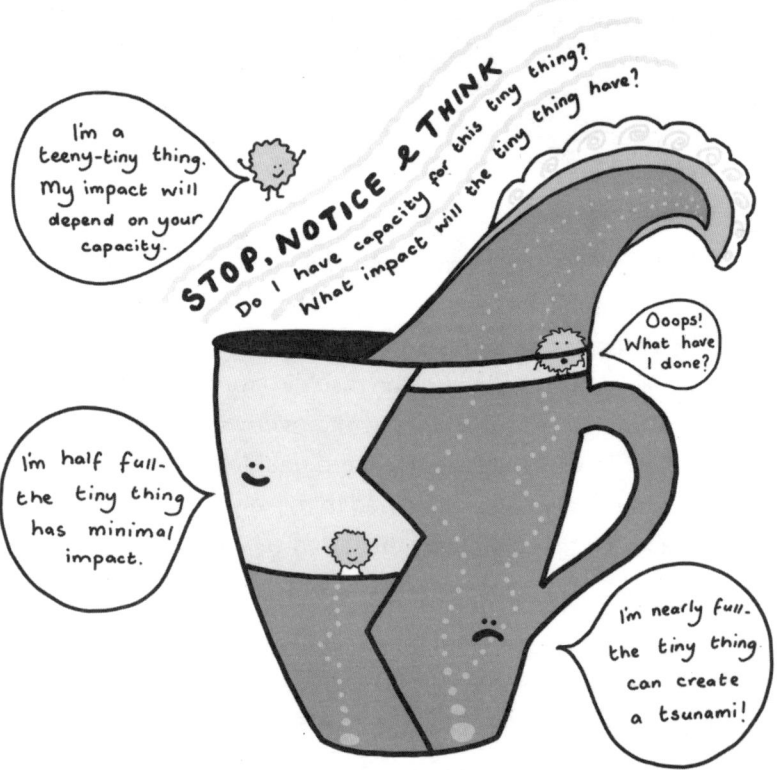

Anti-burnout takeaways

- Caring roles can be rewarding, but they can also be difficult and have physical, cognitive and emotional impacts.
- Often caring roles are unrecognized and undervalued.
- Parental burnout is common and can present slightly differently to standard burnout (see the WHO definition on page 15).
- The impact of paid and unpaid caring increases the risk of burnout. Burnout in carers may also lead to compassion fatigue.
- It's critical to recognize the impact of your caring roles and think about how to manage this.
- The mental load is important to consider in relation to burnout. The mental load is invisible, difficult to quantify, boundaryless and never ending, which means it is constantly filling your capacity cup.
- Women continue to disproportionately carry the mental load, which puts them at greater risk of burnout.
- The mental load is linked to the system around us. Being anti-burnout is about recognizing this so we can alleviate self-blame, shame and personal responsibility.
- We can also take steps to be anti-burnout by taking tiny steps to manage demand and capacity and look after ourselves, while recognizing the impact of the system.

Chapter 8
Different brains and burnout: Why burnout is a neurodiversity issue

My brain is unique. I am not special, though, because your brain is unique too. What's more, your brain is unique to you at this point in time, because you have a slightly different brain to this same time last year, or even last week. There's something rather awe-inspiring about the fact that not one single person in the world has exactly the same brain. Yes, to some extent, there may be similarities in structure and function, but each person's 86 billion neurons and the 100 trillion or so connections between these communicating cells – and I've not even mentioned the rough estimate of 99 billion other supportive cells in your brain – create infinite (or at least a number way larger than my brain can comprehend) possibilities in how they link together and function. When you consider these numbers, it makes perfect sense that every brain can't possibly be the same. Variation is the norm when it comes to brains. I find that a mind-blowing (or perhaps I should say brain-blowing) concept.

Our AMAZING brains

It's fair to say the brain is a complex organ, and what's more, it's so complex we don't fully understand it yet. This is summed up beautifully by a slightly mind-bending quote from the physicist George Pugh's book:[1]

If the human brain were so simple we could understand it, we would be so simple that we couldn't.

Your amazing brain works through connections and predictions to try and keep you functioning well. It's an integral part of your body, with constant communication to and fro. It's the mass of cells through which you filter and make sense of yourself and the world. It anticipates the future and reflects on the past. It creates meaning and stories and art. It stores your past life within your skull. It makes you, you. I am in constant awe of my brain and what it enables me to do. The fact it is helping me think about my brain and yours, transforming those thoughts into sentences and enabling my hands to write these sentences onto the page is amazing. In turn, your amazing brain will form these shapes into words and sentences so you can read them, make sense of them and integrate this information with what's already in your brain. Together, as I type and as you read, we are forming, shifting and strengthening connections, and literally changing our brains. AMAZING.

I sometimes wonder if my awe for my brain, in fact everybody's brain, comes from working with people who find their brain function has changed.* We normally take our brain functioning

---

* I trained and worked in neuropsychology for over 15 years, assessing cognition and working with people who experienced a range of acquired brain injuries.

for granted. Things feel simple to us, not because they are simple, but because our brains are silently working away in complex ways to enable us to feel like tasks are simple. Sometimes it is only when this shifts that we start to realize how complex tasks actually are. Let's take making a cup of tea as an example – a relatively simple task. Or so it seems – until you have a brain injury that affects your cognitive skills and you realize there are multiple complex steps to making a cup of tea. From initiating the task to remembering where the tea bags are, to planning the steps in the correct order, to being able to locate the teapot at the correct point in space, to switching your attention to get the biscuit you prefer from the cupboard (Tunnocks Teacake for me), to being aware of the length of time you have dunked the tea bag, this task is inherently complex. It's a miracle your brain is able to do all of this (and there are many more steps beyond these).

Your cognitive functioning can change in different ways too (sometimes reversible), such as through the result of illness, mental health difficulties, trauma or going through life phases such as pregnancy or menopause. Depression, for example, affects connectivity and creates structural changes in your brain, making it less able to concentrate, more focused on the negative, more exhausting to do tasks and more difficult to learn new information, which shifts again as you recover.[2] And of course burnout creates changes in our brain[3] that affect our cognitive function, how we feel and what we can do. Sometimes it is only when these changes occur that we become aware that our amazing brain has been doing things we have taken for granted, and we start to appreciate the amazing feats our brain is undertaking every single minute of the day.

BURNOUT AND BRAIN FUNCTION

Thinking about brain functioning is important for burnout. Cognitive changes are an outcome of burnout, but our brain and cognitive function are also important factors that may contribute to the development of burnout. You'll already have spotted some of the cognitive changes (which will have been due to underlying brain changes) I had during burnout, including a high level of negative focus, difficulty with planning and selective attention (switching off noise was difficult). In fact, a shift in my cognitive functioning was one of the first symptoms of burnout I spotted: the complete lack of ideas and inability to be creative. This was in stark contrast to some of the ways my brain functioned beforehand, which both helped me and made me me, but which also likely contributed to me becoming burned out. My brain was always busy: I wasn't just juggling a busy life but also a busy brain. I constantly had ideas, things I wanted to do, books I wanted to read, ways I wanted to help and much more. Some of the ways my brain works has some fantastic upsides: I never get bored; I am good at coming up with solutions; I can anticipate and respond to how people feel; I can focus my attention for long periods of time to get things done; I am really enthusiastic about lots of things because I am genuinely interested (I once won a class vote as the most likely person to start a cult, apparently because I had contagious enthusiasm about very random things – or at least that's what they told me!).

But I also recognize that the way my brain functions most likely contributed to my burnout in a number of ways: my ideas often come at night, which is not compatible with sleep; constant ideas and enthusiasm can lead to taking lots on and being too busy; my brain (like my computer!) feels like it has infinite tabs open, which uses lots of energy and is difficult to switch off;

feeling what people feel can be taxing; and maintaining my focus was often at the detriment of taking breaks. Why am I telling you all this about my brain? It's to recognize that while burnout impacts on how our brain functions, how our brain functions can also contribute to burnout.

What about neurodivergent brains?

You may have recognized yourself in some of the ways I described my cognitive function, or your brain may operate in a completely different way (it's unique after all). None of these ways of thinking/processing are better or worse, they are just different, and your brain may function better or worse in different contexts. To me, neurodiversity captures the fact that all our brains function slightly differently. We can all benefit from recognizing which aspect of our own brain functioning can contribute to the risk of us developing burnout, in the context we are in. I do not have a diagnosis to define the way my brain functions, and you do not need a diagnosis to think about your cognitive functioning in this chapter, as we will look at different cognitive functions and how they can contribute to burnout.

However, it is critical we also talk about neurodivergence, which describes when someone's brain processes, learns and functions in a way that differs from what is considered typical* (and I emphasize **considered**, because there is wide variation in how brains function, so it's often unclear what we mean by typical). 'Neurodiverse' is often used as an umbrella term, which includes diagnoses including (but not exclusive to) ADHD,

---

* 'Neurotypical' is defined as thinking and processing in line with societal norms and expectations.

autistic spectrum condition (ASC), dyspraxia and dyslexia. The research tells us that diagnoses of ADHD and ASC (or autism) are associated with increased risk of burnout.[4] However, not everyone who is neurodivergent will have – or want to have – a formal diagnosis. In addition, every neurodivergent person has a completely unique brain – a specific diagnosis does not capture individual complexity. Therefore, not all of the brain factors in this chapter will be relevant to every neurodivergent individual. Also, if you do not have a diagnosis, or do not consider yourself neurodivergent, some of the cognitive and brain aspects I talk about are likely to still be relevant for you. Therefore, I want you to consider how your unique brain operates during this chapter, whether you consider yourself neurodivergent or not, and whether this may be something you need to consider to be anti-burnout.

Some considerations here before we go further. I appreciate that most people will not have worked directly with cognitive functioning and therefore may not have considered their own brain functioning in as much detail as I have. That's okay, just see what resonates with you as you read through this chapter. I will also not be covering all the characteristics of neurodivergent diagnoses here as they are covered extensively elsewhere (you'll find some Further Reading on page 306). I also will not presume to speak from the point of view of neurodivergence: my perspectives are drawn from people I have spoken to, my clinical experience and the research in this area. It's also important to recognize that certain life stages (such as menopause), illnesses and injuries can affect brain functioning, including (but not limited to) cognitive skills such as executive functioning, processing speed, memory and attention, and while I do not cover the impact of these directly in this chapter, it is nonetheless relevant to use this chapter to think about your own brain functioning if it has been affected by other factors, how this impacts you and how this may relate to burnout. Finally, if you are concerned about your brain functioning or cognition, or changes in them, please speak to a healthcare provider who can assess further, help you to understand and advise on suitable supports.

THE WORLD IS DESIGNED FOR OUR IDEA OF NEUROTYPICAL

First, we need to address a central problem and to do this, we need to look at the context around your burnout tree, because this is not normally designed for neurodivergence. I believe this is because we often think we know how the brain should work, and we use this benchmark to set our expectations. These expectations tend to prioritize certain characteristics, such as high organization, compliance with rules, high sociability, emotional containment and focused attention. These expectations are woven into the intrinsic threads of how our society operates and how it expects you to operate within that society. We've already spoken about some examples of societal beliefs and how they apply to burnout generally. However, societal beliefs and expectations may have an even greater impact on a neurodivergent brain: research shows high levels of stress are created by living in a world that doesn't accommodate, understand or support your needs.[5] Living within this context creates extra stress in a multitude of different ways, including (but not limited to):

- Having to/trying to function in a way that does not align with how your brain naturally operates.
- Hiding parts of yourself that do not meet societal expectations.

- Dealing with sensory overload.
- Changes in routine and social demands.
- Experiencing a pervasive lack of awareness, stigma, criticism and discrimination from others.

Not fitting into the world's view of how you should operate can also lead to beliefs that you are somehow different or abnormal, along with self-doubt, internal criticism and a sense of failure, blame and shame.[6] That's a lot of stress! People I have worked with have told me they feel their stress baseline is always at a higher point (and research also supports this[7]) – their capacity cup is always nearly full with these additional demands, which means it doesn't take much more to push into overwhelm. We also know that greater stress that goes on for too long, feels out of control and is difficult to manage can lead to burnout. It's therefore no surprise that neurodivergent brains living in a world that isn't designed for them lead to greater stress and distress and are more likely to burn out as a result.

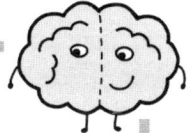

Brian the Brain reflections

Think about the systems around your burnout tree in relation to how your brain functions:

- Considering how your brain operates, which aspects of your environment cause you stress?
- Which aspects do you find emotionally demanding?
- Does the environment around your burnout tree create expectations that you find difficult to meet because of how your brain functions?
- Which aspects of the environment are cognitively demanding or difficult for you to manage?

> - Which, if any, aspects of your functioning do you try to inhibit, hide or mask in the environments in which you exist? How does this impact on you?
> - Are there ways that the environment could work better for you?
> - Are there supports or systems that could be put in place (by yourself or with others) to help manage the system?

NEURODIVERGENT BURNOUT

We had a whistle-stop tour through what burnout is in Chapter 1. However, this burnout definition is mainly focused on research around work. There is increasing recognition that burnout is more common due to certain circumstances or characteristics, and recommendations that we should consider certain sub-types of burnout, including parental burnout and neurodivergent burnout (sometimes defined with a specific diagnosis, such as autism burnout).

Research suggests that neurodivergent burnout may present differently, and the contributory factors and recovery advice may also differ from those traditionally recommended with a neurotypical stance in mind. For a start, research has suggested that neurodivergent burnout is thought to be characterized by additional symptoms compared to traditional burnout. (It's important to note that much of this research has been carried out in people with a specific diagnosis, such as autism or ADHD.) One research study in 2021 by Higgens and colleagues,[8] which aimed to clarify the characteristics of autistic burnout, defined it as:

Different brains and burnout

A severely debilitating condition with onset preceded by fatigue from camouflaging or masking autistic traits, interpersonal interactions, an overload of cognitive input, a sensory environment unaccommodating to autistic sensitivities and/or other additional stressors or change.

You will have spotted the clear differences in factors that lead to burnout, and they also described differences in the symptoms of burnout. Similar to the standard definition, autism burnout was characterized by significant mental and physical exhaustion, but there were also some differences. These included interpersonal withdrawal, reduced functioning, difficulties with executive function and/or increased intensity of autistic traits.

While this is still an emerging research area, current research into neurodivergent burnout generally has suggested that in addition to the classic burnout symptoms such as exhaustion, neurodivergent burnout symptoms may also include: loss of skills, reduced tolerance to environmental stimuli, having to withdraw from being with other people and exacerbated neurodivergent characteristics, such as an increased sensitivity to noise and reduction in executive function abilities.[9]

Brain factors, environmental interactions and burnout

We are now going to consider some brain factors and how they can interact with the environment to create stress, which is relevant to burnout. Being anti-burnout is about being aware of how these factors contribute to stress for you and thinking about what you can do about it. It's also about depersonalizing this and recognizing what the issues actually are and where they are located (such as an environment not designed for you) rather than blaming yourself. Remember to add relevant factors into your burnout tree in the correct location. And a reminder that no cognitive profile is correct or better; everybody has strengths and weaknesses when it comes to cognitive functioning, and we are all different.

1. Masking

This is unintentionally or intentionally suppressing or camouflaging neurodivergent traits and/or aspects of yourself and your identity in order to fit in and manage the expectations of others, to minimize the fear of negative repercussions.

Studies that look at masking suggest it is a common and consistent behaviour in people who are neurodivergent, and it occurs in other groups of people where there is more stigma, such as those with mental illness and brain injury. Research highlights that for many people, this is such an inherent behaviour that 'masking is life'.[10] It is effortful and uses energy and cognitive resources; you constantly self-monitor, suppress natural responses and initiate alternative responses. All this uses up capacity and energy and can contribute to baseline levels of stress.

Research indicates that masking can be exhausting and have a mental health impact, as well as leading to loss of identity and even an experience of grief, as you feel you cannot be yourself.[11] Feeling impelled to hide aspects of yourself can also be associated with shame and have a significant emotional impact. Masking is thought to be a key factor leading to higher levels of burnout in neurodivergent populations because of the ongoing stress and effort of masking itself and the impact it can have.[12]

2. Perspective disconnect

Studies have suggested that neurodivergent people often express having their concerns ignored and feeling like they are not being believed.[13] Concerns can be misunderstood, dismissed or trivialized, and the person receives a lack of empathy from other people, which can be stressful and have negative emotional and practical consequences, leading to increased likelihood of masking. I have also seen this occur with brain injury and other mental and physical illnesses that affect functioning, which can result in people feeling devalued, doubting themselves, self-blaming and self-shaming.

3. Discrimination and stigma

Any form of discrimination and stigma creates stress for our tree branches to hold, leading to a greater likelihood of masking as a coping mechanism to avoid negative consequences. Greater discrimination across a range different populations is associated with higher levels of burnout as it causes high levels of stress.[14]

4. Lack of support and barriers to it

A critical factor in anyone's burnout tree is the social support that they receive, which helps build strong roots and protect against burnout. However, when you have additional needs, you may need additional practical and emotional support yet may find it difficult to recognize when you need it and where to get it from. There can also be significant barriers to accessing formal support, including long waiting lists or financial limitations, or the supports may just not exist. While not having the support can weaken your tree, multiple aspects of trying to access the support you need can also be frustrating and exhausting, therefore adding stressors to your branches. These stressors include: having to advocate for yourself; sharing your personal story; the difficulties of navigating the care system; feeling isolated and devalued by society because the support doesn't exist.

5. Cognitive load and effort

Cognitive load is the amount of information your brain is carrying at any one time. A constantly high load uses your energy and can deplete you. Cognitive load can be due to both external demands and internal factors, such as attention capacity. People with neurodivergence tend to report higher cognitive load and more frequent overload, which can add to stress and impact on functioning. Cognitive effort is the amount of cognitive resources you are having to use to complete a task. In people with neurodivergence, certain tasks (such as planning, organizing and socializing) may take additional effort and resources, which can be exhausting. The extra cognitive effort tasks require may lead to compensatory behaviours that can contribute to burnout, such as staying late at work to catch up. The more cognitive effort tasks take, the more energy your brain is guzzling, leading to greater exhaustion and depletion.

6. I'm an empath, get me out of here!

Empathy is the ability to understand or share the emotions or experiences of others and react to their internal state. It can be divided into **cognitive empathy**, which is the intellectual ability to understand the perspective of others; and **emotional empathy**, a response to how others feel.

In my clinical work, people with neurodivergence often describe experiencing emotions deeply as well as sensitivity to how other people feel, and there are many personal descriptions of this[15] plus some supporting research, suggesting higher levels of emotional empathy in autism.[16] While high levels of empathy are often regarded as a positive trait, they can have a downside: you may experience heightened sensitivity to suffering, which can be exhausting, emotionally demanding and deplete your resources. It's no surprise that research suggests that high levels of empathy may contribute to burnout.[17] It may also lead to behaviours that can contribute to burnout in themselves, such as over-involvement, feeling compelled to help and difficulty setting boundaries.

7. Sensory processing

Sensory processing sensitivity is being sensitive to external or internal sensory stimuli. This might mean you are more distracted or even overwhelmed by certain textures or have difficulty switching off from certain sounds or visual stimuli. This can result in high stress levels and overwhelm, and you may become overstimulated, for example in busy spaces. If your capacity cup is already full (perhaps you are stressed or working under high demands), then sensory sensitivity can increase. Again, it's probably not surprising that research indicates that sensory processing sensitivity may contribute to burnout, and that sensory overload can increase during burnout in the neurodivergent population.[18]

8. Emotion processing

Just like our brains are all different, how we experience and process emotions differs across different people, and emotional processing differences can occur as part of a neurodivergent presentation.[19] Emotions can hit harder and last longer for some people. It may also be more difficult for some people to notice, monitor, understand and modify their emotions. Emotional lability, when strong emotions appear in quick succession, sometimes not consistent with the context, can occur with neurodivergence, brain injury and certain mental and physical health presentations. It's also common for heightened anxiety-type symptoms to occur more spontaneously with certain illnesses and conditions, including menopause. This can result in emotions being stronger, more stressful, more difficult to manage and feeling more out of control, which can have a greater cognitive and emotional impact. It may also be diffiicult to notice emotions, so we don't spot them and attend to them when we need to or ask for additional support. This is consistent with research that indicates that some people with a neurodivergent profile will not notice they are burned out until much later on in its course.[20]

9. Executive functioning factors

Executive function is the manager and coordinator of the brain: it will help you to initiate, plan, organize and prioritize tasks, switch between tasks and choose which information to filter in and out. Aspects of executive functioning are often highlighted as differences in people with neurodivergence. We won't go through the whole list of functions here, but here are some that are particularly relevant when it comes to burnout:

- **Mental flexibility** – This is the ability to be flexible and adapt to new information, changes or unplanned events. If mental flexibility is more difficult, then it can be harder for your brain to take in and process new information and adapt to changes. Tasks requiring these skills can be more effortful and cognitively demanding. This can mean that while you enjoy familiarity and routine, change is hard and overwhelming, or you can get stuck in particular ways of thinking or acting.
- **Planning and organizing** – If planning and organizing is more effortful, it can be more difficult to manage your

time, to prioritize and to balance different elements of your life, which can result in feeling stressed, overwhelmed and out of control. Moreover, from clinical experience, we tend to put these skills on a pedestal, and they relate to employability, efficiency and worth. If you look at job descriptions, they are normally on there somewhere. When these skills don't come naturally, we can feel inadequate, blame ourselves and feel like there is something inherently wrong with us. Difficulties with planning and organizing (and other executive functioning abilities) can also lead to procrastination, as initiating or planning a task is difficult, so outcomes feel hard to achieve and require additional effort.[21]

10. Attention factors

- **Focused attention** – This can keep us on task; however, hyper-focused attention can mean we stay on-task for too long, don't take breaks and keep going until the task is finished.[22] This can be exhausting and stressful for our brain and can also have a detrimental impact on other aspects of our life, which may be neglected. We may also fail to take the breaks our brain and body require to re-energize.
- **Impulsivity** – This is the tendency to jump in quickly without thinking. It can result in starting things without finishing others, or taking on tasks without thinking about the impact. This can lead to having many tasks on the go at once, taking on more than we can manage, which in turn leads to cognitive overload, overwhelm and stress.

Different brains and burnout

- **Hyperactivity** – This is about being constantly active, getting bored easily, being restless and having difficulty switching off. It's easy to think how this could be related to burnout, as we may stay in a busy, switched-on mode for long periods of time and have difficulty slowing down or switching off to relax. It can also lead to constant rushing, which can be stressful. Getting bored easily might lead to taking on more tasks than we have capacity for.
- **Distractibility** – This is about being easily distracted from a task, either by external or internal stimuli. Being more distractible can lead to greater cognitive strain and load and can impact task completion. This, in turn, can impact work performance and mean you take more time to complete tasks, which you may then have to catch up on.

What helps a neurodivergent brain be anti-burnout?

When speaking with my neurodivergent friends about this, a constant theme came up: traditional recommendations around wellbeing or how to manage burnout often don't work for them. This advice tends to be about gradually building up activities or increasing social contact, when actually they just need to shut down or have time alone. This is critical, as well-meaning support that is incompatible with the needs of autistic adults may prolong or worsen episodes of autistic burnout.[23] In addition, research suggests that for neurodivergent people to be anti-burnout and recover from burnout, it's often critical to look at the immediate environment in which a person is operating, and that might be about other people making changes rather than the person themselves.[24]

This might include training managers and colleagues in neurodivergence, with the aim of shifting expectations and increasing understanding, acceptance and compassion. It can also include practical adaptations to the environment to make it more suitable for the person, making reasonable adjustments in response to their individual needs and support. In addition, recognizing that there are high levels of shame and blame through living in a world that doesn't fully understand neurodiversity means that connecting with other people to share experiences and ideas and find support can be helpful.

Basically, to become anti-burnout we need a tectonic cultural shift from assuming that everybody's brain works similarly to understanding and valuing brain differences and building the world around these. But there are also things that can be done now proactively so you can be anti-burnout in your own life. Self-awareness of the factors contributing to burnout and proactive management around these can also support you to be anti-burnout, and that is what the next exercise focuses on.

Anti-burnout Exercise 17: Your brain and burnout

This exercise is about recognizing which of your brain characteristics may feed into your stress levels and risk of burnout, then thinking about how to manage this, within the boundaries of what is realistic and possible. For example, you may recognize that masking feeds into your burnout tree as it creates additional stress, but it may not feel safe to unmask in your current work circumstances. However, you may feel able to speak to a few close friends

Different brains and burnout

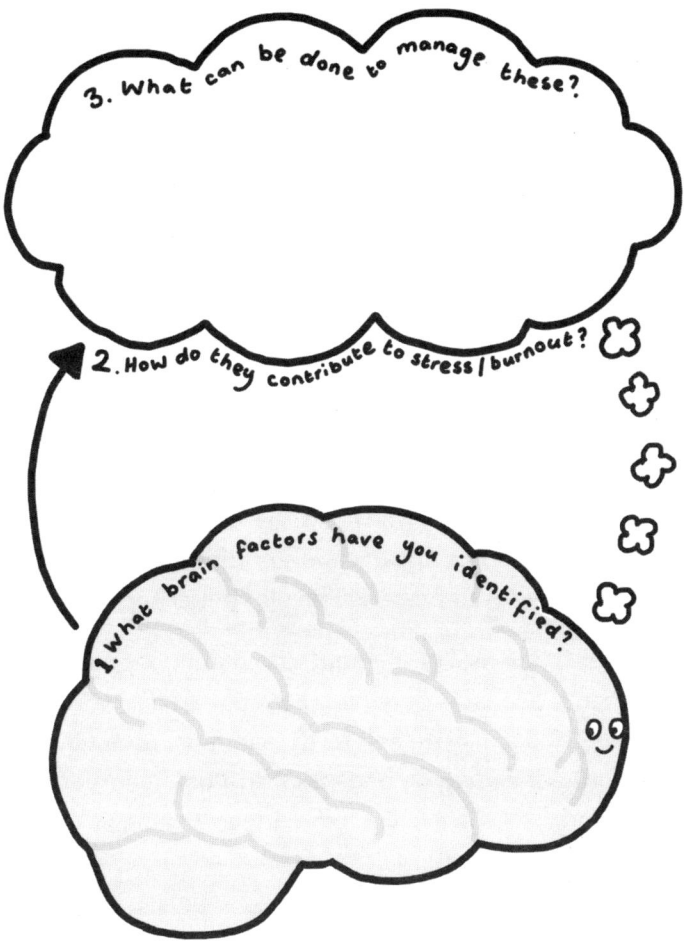

or acknowledge the stress this causes in work, so you can plan something to decompress afterwards.

Use the brain image to think about your relevant brain factors and current environmental challenges and how these create, or interact to create, stress.

Next consider how these factors and challenges can best be supported to manage stress. There are multiple possible ways to do this – what works for you depends on your own preferences and situation. This is not about changing you as person – you are quite alright how you are. The solutions here will predominantly be environmental. For example:

- Prompts to remind you to take a break rather than hyper-focusing.
- Reducing environmental distractions.
- Removing sensory overload.
- Accessing support, which may be for yourself or to support workplaces, schools or other people to understand your presentation and better support you.

The best solutions, I have found, come from people who have had personal experience sharing what has worked for them, and it may be helpful to read more about this (see Further Reading on page 306) and/or join forums or networks, so you can find other ideas that may work for you.

If you are wondering after reading this chapter that you might be neurodivergent and would like this to be assessed further, speak to your GP or another relevant healthcare professional.

Anti-burnout takeaways

- Everybody's brain functions slightly differently.
- Many environments are designed for what we consider neurotypical, meaning that they can be difficult for people whose cognitive style differs from this.
- Some brain styles may increase the risk of burnout, including neurodivergence. This is due to the impact on the person's life and is linked to their environment.
- There are a number of brain-related factors that may increase stress and therefore potentially contribute to a higher risk of burnout.
- These include factors in the environment in which your brain exists, such as lack of understanding and barriers to support.
- They also include cognitive factors, such as empathy, attention and executive function styles.
- It's important to recognize brain factors that are creating stress and adding to the weight on your burnout tree branches.
- You can find ways to manage and support these brain factors. Many of these supports will be environmental to help you cope and manage better, as YOU are not the problem!

PART 3
Relighting Your Fire: What To Do If You Are Burned Out

Chapter 9

The emotional impact of burnout

So, you've burned out (hey, who hasn't!). Burnout can be a lonely place: it can feel like we are the only one lost in an isolated arctic outpost, from which there's no escape and where it's too cold to ever relight our fire. All our perceived personal failures and mistakes have led to us taking a one-way path to this desolated and dismal place, where we will languish in our own shame forever, in a frozen zombie state. However, the reality is somewhat different. You have come to a place of togetherness, where many people will arrive at some point (in this chapter we'll meet some of the ex-zombies who have been here before). But it's not an outpost: it's a collective human experience; it's a community; it's a reaction to the weight of life that many of us have to hold; it's a perfectly normal dip on that path of life on which we all travel. Life is a series of problems we need to solve, and this is no different; it's just another part of life we need to navigate. It feels like there is no escape, but we just need to find the pathways out of the snowy mist, back to ourselves and our lives again, or perhaps a different version we build intentionally. Our burnout tree may feel irreparably crushed by the weight, but its capacity for growth is still there, resting through its arctic winter and regaining energy, waiting until it is safe to grow again, establish new roots and develop fresh leaves and stronger branches. I found Katherine May's quote, from her book *Wintering*, comforting during my burnout:

> *Life meanders like a path through the woods. We have seasons where we flourish and seasons where the leaves fall from us, revealing our bare bones. Given time, they grow again.*[1]

There are many paths out of burnout. However, in the arctic depths of winter, holed up in this outpost, getting out can feel challenging, and there are multiple barriers in our way. Finding the ways out can be difficult and feel effortful, and (like most change) the first step is especially tough, as we step into the unknown, away from our norm, as this arctic outpost has become. All of us, even with the best intentions (and even with psychology training), unintentionally do things that trap us further. The isolation can feel strangely safe – we start to become established in our discomfort. Conversely, the pathways out can feel treacherous – maybe we will make another mistake and take the wrong path out, stumbling into somewhere darker than where we are already? As we look out from this outpost with burned-out eyes, the pathways out are unclear, the world feels full of overwhelming risk, and more change might just make us feel even more broken.

Burnout has emotional, physical and situational repercussions. Learning to understand and respond to these in ways that feel safe and manageable (and don't just make us sink further) are how we locate the paths out. We can start to take gradual steps along these routes and find ways to avoid the barriers and traps that tell us we should stay. Although the outpost may feel safer than the pathways out, this is an illusion. Staying should only ever be temporary, because this is a fragile place: the zombies can never relight their fires in this perpetual cold. Stay too long and you might just become frozen in time. Being anti-burnout is about finding the paths out and daring to step on them. By doing this we move through the arctic winter to start to thaw, grow again, relight our fire and maybe even build back stronger. Let's start our journey.

7 Emotional pathways out of burnout

Emotional Pathway 1: Legitimizing your experience

One of the issues that I have seen persistently throughout my clinical career is that we doubt and invalidate our experiences and illnesses, particularly if there isn't a clear physical manifestation or marker of them. In burnout, this creates a trap that keeps us stuck.

Time to meet out first ex-zombie, Zoe, who was a nurse in a busy ward. She had high standards and was exceptionally caring. After her 12-hour shifts, she could barely function and spent her time between shifts sleeping and watching daytime TV (enough to depress anybody, she told me) because she had no energy until her next shift. Like me, she was at the burnout arctic outpost for quite some time before she recognized she was there. When I first met her, she told me there was nothing wrong with her, she just needed to learn to be more motivated, focused and resilient. She believed she wasn't as good a nurse as her colleagues and berated herself for being lazy and letting people down. To assuage the resulting guilt, she took on

The emotional impact of burnout

extra shifts, working more overtime, which resulted in feeling even more exhausted in between shifts. Not recognizing she was burned out was keeping her stuck. Failing to recognize burnout and just keeping on going is the opposite of being anti-burnout: it's the burnout trap. It traps us into believing we should just push on through, we should do better, that we should negate and hide how we feel, that no one will believe us (why would they when we don't even believe ourselves?). This keeps us in a perpetual cycle of burnout, stuck in the outpost.

We may not see indicators in our brain or body, and there is no clear diagnostic test, however this doesn't make burnout any less real than any other illness or experience. We know that there are multiple physiological changes that occur in burnout, which we go into in detail in the next chapter. These underlying changes will explain many of the symptoms we see in our zombie army, including perpetually increased threat responses, exhaustion and increased levels of illnesses. Just because you can't see them, doesn't mean they aren't real. How you feel and the shift in your functioning is your body and brain shouting to you, loud and clear, that they are injured and need to recover. Like any injury or illness, you need to rest and recuperate. The first step to enable you to do this is to recognize and legitimize what you are experiencing. For Zoe, it was only by recognizing her symptoms and putting a name to them (she also visited her GP), as well as understanding the underlying physiology and why this had developed, that she was able to legitimize how she felt, recognize that she needed to take steps to recover and was able to start down the pathways out of burnout.

Legitimizing your experiences is being able to recognize that you are experiencing something real and tangible – it is not something imagined or existing only in your mind. Burnout is an injury that requires treatment, that takes time to heal from and needs real, tangible steps to recover. Validating what you are experiencing has to be the first pathway out of burnout. Once you can start to say with confidence (even just to yourself) 'I AM BURNED OUT', pathways and possibilities start to open up before you to help you heal and recover. Even just the recognition itself starts to thaw your burnout arctic slightly and fans the flames that felt impossible to reignite. You shift from using strategies that are freezing you in perpetuity, to pathways that start to thaw you out.

What might legitimizing your experience look like?

1. **Validation:** For many people it's getting validation through a medical expert/healthcare professional that what they are experiencing is burnout. I would recommend this, as it also helps rule out other possible causes and provides a clear, confirmed name/definition to capture and communicate your experience. A healthcare professional can also help you to access treatment and/or support if you require time off work.
2. **Therapy:** Seeking professional services can be a further way to legitimize your experiences and help you make sense of your story and the factors contributing to it. It can help you understand how you got here, what's keeping you stuck and find pathways forward in a supported environment. This is particularly helpful if you recognize that difficult or traumatic past experiences have been contributary factors to your burnout.

3. **Understanding:** Taking time to understand your symptoms and factors contributing to their development can also be helpful. You can do this using the burnout tree in Chapter 2, or you may wish to list your symptoms and talk them through with someone else or draw a timeline of your experiences/symptoms and how they have developed/changed over time.

Emotional Pathway 2: Hold on to hope

Please note, if you are feeling hopeless, are unable to see any future or are starting to think people would be better without you or about harming yourself, seek immediate help through a healthcare professional.

Being in the arctic-outpost depths of burnout can feel hopeless – is there really a pathway out? You feel frozen, unable to do anything. There appears to be no way forward, that your flame will never reignite. You've tried so many things that don't work, now you feel helpless to do anything: what's the point if all the energy you muster to do something makes you feel worse? To start to even see through the fog, we need hope. Hope that there are ways out but also that enables us to sit in the outpost for a while, so we can gather the energy to go down those pathways. Initially, when I recognized I was burned out, I needed to retreat and wrap a blanket around me in the tundra to warm myself slightly and give myself a little energy before I was able to take any more steps. To allow myself to do this, I needed hope that things could change; but holding this belief is hard for a zombie brain with little energy, overrun with an army of negative ninjas telling you the opposite. Hope lets us sit still, knowing there is a path forward. Hope can enable us to take gradual steps out and keep us going even when the steps falter or we misstep (which we will).

The first step is realizing that hope is not something that is lost in this arctic outpost – many zombies have passed through here before. The decline you have experienced is not irreversible and although it may feel dormant right now, growth is still possible. Your brain and body can heal and repair and can even grow back stronger. Life may feel ruptured, but you can build something better. You are not helpless in getting out, you have agency to take the steps forward. Even better, you do not have to do it alone, as there is an army of current and ex-zombies to help you. Getting here is not an unusual or abnormal occurrence: most people pass through their version of an arctic winter at some point in their life, whether through burnout or other experiences that make our lives take unexpected dips and detours. Getting here is just life, and being here is just human. Finding hope and building back from a dark place where it feels like there are no paths forward is one of the greatest skills humans have, which we are all capable of and can all support each other in doing.

Anti-burnout Exercise 18: Finding hope

Hope is something you can find, cultivate and build on. You can find it in many ways: through recognizing the humanness of your experiences, from hearing stories of ex-zombies or sharing your own experiences, remembering how you got through tough times before. You can seek hope in the words and connections with

The emotional impact of burnout

others or through their comfort or support. You can capture glimmers of hope when you fleetingly spot signs of the pathways out or find pockets of joy or regrowth. Once you find it, you need to cultivate it and build on it by holding on to it, reminding yourself of it and not letting it go. Think about how you will hold on to hope using the image below.

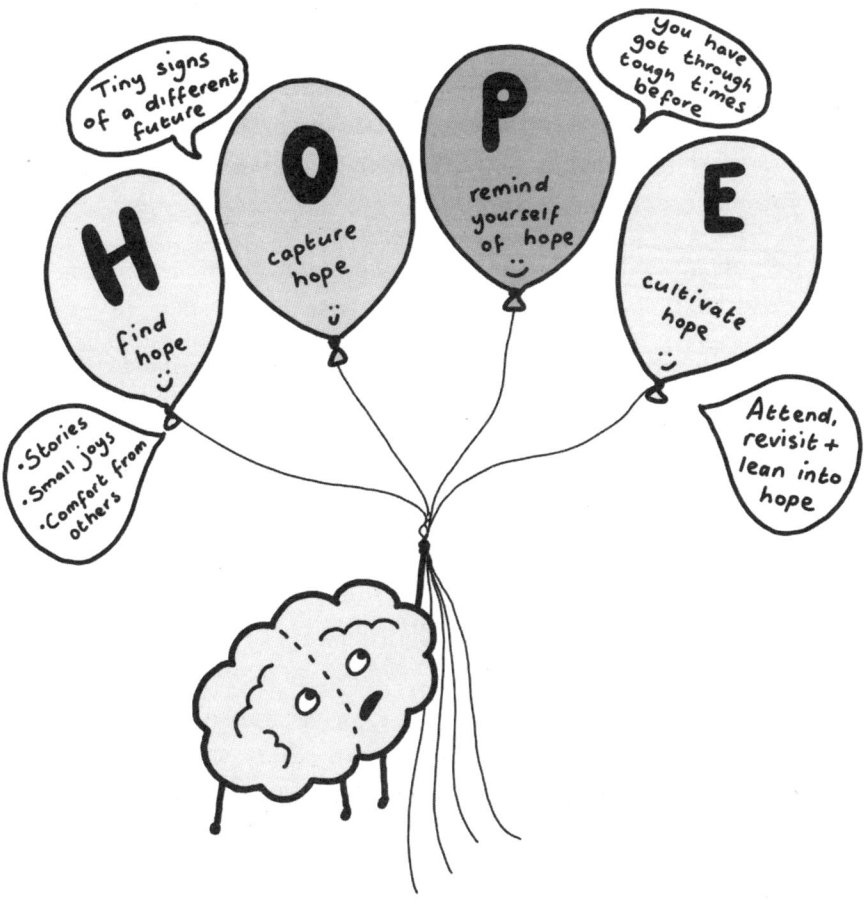

Emotional Pathway 3: Softening your shame

PLEASE NOTE: If shame is a deeply held belief or related to traumatic experiences, this process is often best supported within a safe therapeutic space with a trained professional.

Shame is an intrinsic part of many illnesses, particularly those we can't see; those which we have more difficulty legitimizing to ourselves; those which society still places blame and personal responsibility on the sufferer due to historical beliefs (mental illness being the clear example here). Shame tells us there is something fundamentally wrong with us, that we are responsible, that we have done something to bring this upon ourselves. It takes our experiences, dismisses any external contributory factors and instead locates the problem inside us, as something about us. It's not something that has happened to you: you are the error.

Burnout takes shame by the hand and invites it in. When resources are lowered, shame creeps in past our defences and settles in unchallenged. Or perhaps shame has always been there – a force we thought we'd overcome, but its tentacles rise again from the deep as we have less energy and resources to keep it down and our rapidly multiplying negative ninjas grab a loudspeaker and amplify its voice. Obviously, it's your fault you have become lost in this arctic tundra, and it's a fundamental personal flaw that has withered you to a zombie. Your very symptoms of burnout are an indication of your worth and moral value.

Let's meet another ex-zombie, Zac, a construction worker. He told me he should consider himself lucky as he had just survived a round of redundancies. He told me he had to be strong or he would be a let-down to his colleagues, friends and the company. If they found out he wasn't coping they would think he was useless at his job and they had made the wrong choice to keep him on. This shame was the burnout trap for Zac: he hid how he felt and it stopped him seeking support or sharing concerns. As a result, his shame grew and took greater control. Once Zac named his shame, we were able draw it out and recognize what it was telling him. He was able to step back and look at it from a different perspective and replace it with what he truly believed. Through understanding why he had burned out, by speaking to his family and manager (who were far more understanding than he anticipated) and by joining an online support group, he developed a more compassionate narrative. This reminded him that burnout was a common experience, not something shameful or abnormal about him.

We've already seen that shame is insidious – it creates hidden networks in our brain so it can implant its ideas and feelings into our minds. Shame likes to hide, to make you believe that it's not there. If you can't see it, you can't do anything about it, which means it can grow and grow, until its mycelian network completes a hostile takeover of your brain. Shame knows if you spot it; if you know it's there, you can shrink it. Bringing shame into the light and into your awareness, exposing it and looking at it with a different perspective (outside of our naturally subjective inner world) starts to separate it from you, to objectify it and soften it into something more mouldable and manageable.

Anti-burnout Exercise 19: Shame hide-and-seek

Before we can soften shame, we need to seek it out, which can be hard because shame wants to hide from us. Try the steps on page 200.

1. **Don't let shame hide!** Seek and name it: You've met my shame, Shane. What character, name, shape, form or colour would your shame have? Defining shame in a way that works for you can help you spot when it is speaking and externalize it. Shame is something that happens, a belief that can shift, rather than being intrinsically about you.
2. **Put shame in the spotlight:** We need to bring shame out into the open so you can expose it for what it really is: a thought, an outdated belief, an old story resurfacing. You will most likely start to notice patterns of what shame tells you. These normally tap into societal expectations, messages that we have been given or perhaps things you have been directly told throughout your life. Seeing shame in this stark light can be enough to help you see the ridiculousness of what shame is saying. You may be able to stand back and observe, 'That's shame speaking again, telling me his old stories. It's not fact, it's just a thought that shame wants me to believe.'
3. **Soften your shame into something more mouldable:** I imagine the process of softening shame like finding an old bit of playdough, peeling back the hard outer layers to reveal the vulnerable inner and then warming the remainder in your hands to comfort and soften it so it becomes more pliable. It might still be there, but its sharp edges have gone and it is less likely to hurt you. There are many ways to soften shame. These include:
   - Self-compassion and receiving compassion
   - Being vulnerable and sharing what shame tells you
   - Finding common experiences

- Recognizing that what you are experiencing is not something fundamentally wrong with you, it just part of human experience.

Speaking your shame aloud in a safe, supported place/space or hearing other people speak about their shame or similar experiences enables us to release it out of its hard hiding place and soften it into something more malleable. See Further Reading on page 306 for a list of resources I found helpful to soften shame around burnout, including books and podcasts.

Emotional Pathway 4: Beware of bouncing back

Dear burnout zombies: This is a public health warning about the toxic nature of wellbeing culture, which idolizes resilience and personal responsibility and tells us to do the work to get better. We are told that 'wellbeing' is something that can be attained through working harder – a goal in itself, an additional unrealistic THERE. And if wellbeing is down to personal responsibility, what does that say? It says that if you fail, yes, of course, it's your fault.

We all love a redemptive recovery story where adversity is overcome to get to a better place. We all want to find the solutions to distress and to bounce back. But this can be a trap in burnout that makes you rush down illusionary pathways to a mythical THERE, to only fall back deeper into the arctic outpost and extinguish more of your flames. Before you set off down any pathway, you need to pause, rest and allow yourself to be there. You may feel broken, but the reality is that distress and suffering is a part of life we need to acknowledge, sit with and understand, not overpower and overcome. Rushing to bounce back makes us work hard to get to a place to stifle or deny this suffering. Recovery is a gradual process that involves recognizing the pain. It requires consideration to find the right route out and patience, as there will be missteps, pauses and pain on the pathways out. To build back sustainably it requires as much dismantling of beliefs, behaviours and surrounding structures as it does building.

Research tells us recovery from burnout can take time, maybe even years, and have ups and downs.[2] If we see this with a realistic lens, then we remove the pressure to bounce back. We break down unrealistic standards and we allow ourselves to feel bad and accept support. We recognize the realistic steps forward and don't berate ourselves for the inevitable steps back. We can be patient with ourselves and celebrate small, slow steps and accept that feeling bad is not a failure, it's just part of life. If you allow yourself to pause among the pieces, truly understand them, dismantle some further and then start to gradually and intentionally build back, with the knowledge that it is not a linear process, then you can build back stronger in a more sustainable way.

Brian the Brain reflections

- Are you pressurizing yourself to bounce back?
- Are you telling yourself you need to do it all on your own?
- Do you view resilience as a personal responsibility?
- Do you believe that feeling bad/suffering is a personal failure?
- How can you give yourself permission to feel bad?

The emotional impact of burnout

- How can you be patient with yourself while you recover?
- How can you allow yourself to learn from your experiences rather than rush back to where you were before?
- How can you set realistic expectations for recovery?

Emotional Pathway 5: Don't be a sh*t to yourself

You might call it your inner critic, your brain bully, negative self-talk. Entrepreneur and author Mo Gawdat calls his Becky.[3] Whatever you call it, we are referring to the critical voice with which you speak to yourself; your private monologue (visual or verbal); your inevitably subjective inner voice that goes with you through life, chattering to you, berating you, sometimes going as far as hating you (if this is the case, time to get a therapist). Not everyone's inner monologue is critical, but many of them are. Certainly, this has been a key theme throughout my twenty-plus years as a clinical psychologist – people berate themselves constantly and this can impact negatively on mental health and be a barrier to getting better.

If you have reached burnout, I would hazard a guess that your inner monologue falls on the critical side, and this may have been a contributory factor to your burnout. A constant brain bully worsens stressors and creates even more for you to hold. Unfortunately (due to the impact of burnout on your brain) at the very time you need to reduce stress and need extra care and compassion, Becky, Belinda, Blake, Bentley or whatever you call your inner critic grabs a microphone to shout louder in an even more critical, nasty tone.

The Anti-Burnout Book

I sometimes think it's a design flaw in our brain that when we need compassion most, when our brain is already blasted by life, we turn on ourselves and blast it some more. We are often total sh*ts to ourselves. Everyone else copes, why can't you? What's wrong with YOU? You are weak, broken, useless, a waste of space. I feel stressed just writing this, so imagine how much stress this constant criticism in your head creates? But you probably don't have to imagine – I bet it's been happening while reading this book. We can be supportive colleagues, friends and family members, but our inner voice will not display these characteristics to ourselves, in fact, quite the opposite. It beats us up for making mistakes, for feeling bad, tired and overwhelmed, for the symptoms of burnout, for being imperfect humans in a complex world.

Self-compassion can be a powerful antidote, and it's a skill we could all do with learning. But when we have frozen malfunctioning zombie brains, the lack of energy and resources mean that it's difficult to even do the basics, and full-on self-compassion just seems impossible. We need simple techniques to shift from sh*t to cheerleader, and we may need support from other brains to help us (social compassion can be very powerful too). So, tune in, turn it down and transform your inner critic. Put it in the phone booth, give it a cloak and see what emerges: maybe a full Clark Kent critic to Superman cheerleader transformation – or maybe we'll just neutralize it to a more manageable level.

The emotional impact of burnout

Anti-burnout Exercise 20: Tune in, turn it down and transform your inner critic

Anytime you start being a sh*t to yourself, tune in, turn it down (pop your inner critic in the phone booth) and transform your inner critic into your inner cheerleader instead.

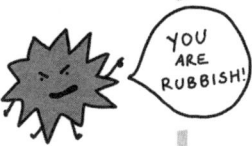

1. **Tune in:** Spot when you are being nasty to yourself. If you like, you can name your inner critic and imagine what it looks or sounds like. It might be the same voice as shame, but it might be something completely different. When I asked on social media what your inner critic looked like, I got a brilliant response – from a patronizing pike to an omnipresent octopus. This can be fun and help you recognize when that voice appears.

2. **Turn it down:** Pop your critic in the phone booth so we can't hear it so loudly. There are many other ways you can turn it down – think of some if you can.

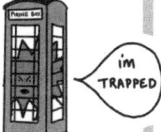

3. **Transform it:** This is where your inner critic dons a cloak and transforms into your inner cheerleader (or at least something more neutral if you can't muster the energy to cheer). Let your inner cheerleader (or just not-so-nasty) character emerge. It speaks to you in a way you need to be spoken to, or how you speak to someone you care about. What does the new character look like and how does it sound? What does it say? My own personal cheerleader is a chutney jar (random, I know). Cheerleader-chutney takes on my friends' voices and reminds me of what they would say to me, and what I would say to them in a similar situation.

Emotional Pathway 6: Help your negative ninjas to retreat

We know that every brain has a negativity bias – the brain is more likely to notice and remember bad things and has a stronger, longer-lasting physiological response to them.[4] This is why one not-so-positive comment stands out in your mind over the thousand neutral or nice comments you receive the same day. This design means we all have negative ninjas working inside our brain to predict, spot, amplify and hold on to the negative. This can feel bad, but the negative ninjas are an evolutionary design to help us spot threat so we can survive.

If we could look inside those burnout zombies' brains, we would see that the negative ninjas have been gathering strength and are rising as an army to swarm their host brain. This evolutionary mechanism, designed to be helpful, has gone into overdrive. Studies of people experiencing burnout have suggested they have greater startle responses and more difficulty downregulating difficult emotions[5] – basically, bad things make them respond even more and stay with them for even longer. When you experience long-term stress, changes in your brain mean you are even more likely to predict, spot and remember negatives. This makes sense: in order to survive through tough times, we need to be able to predict and respond quicker to threat. However, these brain changes can get us stuck in burnout. Our brain becomes so threat-sensitive that it is difficult to move out of it. Not only are your ninjas highlighting the negatives like they are supposed to, but there are also so many ninjas that the negatives become overwhelming, and the army is kicking any positives away before they've even had a chance to enter your attention.

The emotional impact of burnout

The best way to counteract this negative-ninja army is to open your attention to the good stuff. Ex-zombie Zoe was convinced that she was rubbish at her job and at her life and told me all the things that had gone wrong. With gentle, intentional shifts of attention, gradually she was able to let the good stuff in: the patient who thanked her for listening, the positive feedback from her supervisor, the flowers she had grown in the garden, the laughs she shared in messages with her friends. These things had always been there, but the negative ninjas stopped her seeing them. By letting them into her attention they grew and formed memories that lingered, and future good things become more apparent.

We might feel like we want to karate-chop our negative ninjas where it hurts, but actually this just makes them fight back harder (they are far more skilled and practised at this fighting game). A gentler approach is required. If you can intentionally attend to and let just a little bit of the good stuff into your brain space, then your negative ninjas will retreat. We can never get rid of them entirely (and we don't want to, as they have a job to do), but with time, instead of kicking all joy out, they return to their normal job of keeping you safe.

> **Anti-burnout Exercise 21:**
> **Return the negative ninjas to base camp**
>
> There are lots of ways to gently let the good stuff in, to help those negative ninjas retreat. Begin gently – it's not another big 'to do'. Try to do at least one teeny-tiny thing daily, even just for a few minutes. See examples overleaf.

- At the end of the day, write down three things that made you feel good or went well.
- Take pictures of things that make you feel good and store them in a folder on your phone. Open it up when you feel bad.
- Reflect on what you are proud of.
- Stop and notice something joyful in your environment – it might be a beautiful flower you grew or your children's artwork.

If you don't manage any of these things, just try again tomorrow. Because even a bit of gentle refocusing on the good has a powerful retreat effect on your negative ninjas.

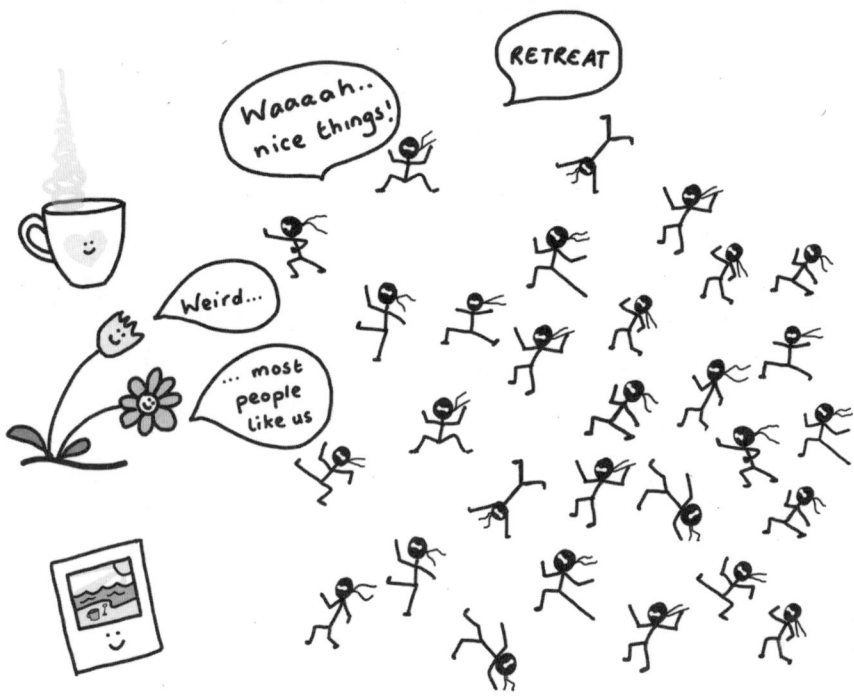

THE DREADED DIFFICULT EMOTIONS
Emotional Pathway 7: Give emotions some space and let them guide you

Yikes, difficult emotions. I really wish they didn't exist. They can make us feel rubbish, so of course we want to get rid of them. Sadly, we can't, as emotions, even the tough ones, are a fundamental and required part of brain functioning. Difficult emotions are part and parcel of burnout, and the more we push them away, ironically the more stress this adds to your burnout tree. If we trap, squash or bottle them, they stay with us, fight back and grow. Giving emotions space feels counterintuitive, but they need space to be able to move on.

Being anti-burnout is about learning to relate to these difficult emotions in a helpful way. Rather than using them as further fuel for blame and shame, it's about identifying them as indicators of your need, for comfort, compassion, space, time or support. Rather than interpreting them as something inherently wrong with you, it's about recognizing that they are normal brain responses to life.

You don't always have to dig around and find the answer to why you are feeling this way; sometimes you can and sometimes you can't. But you can always use those emotions as a compass to help navigate your responses. Ignoring this emotional compass keeps you stuck. However, if you respond to your emotions with space and compassion, and let your emotional compass (how you feel), guide you and your actions, then they can help navigate us to the paths out and guide us along them.

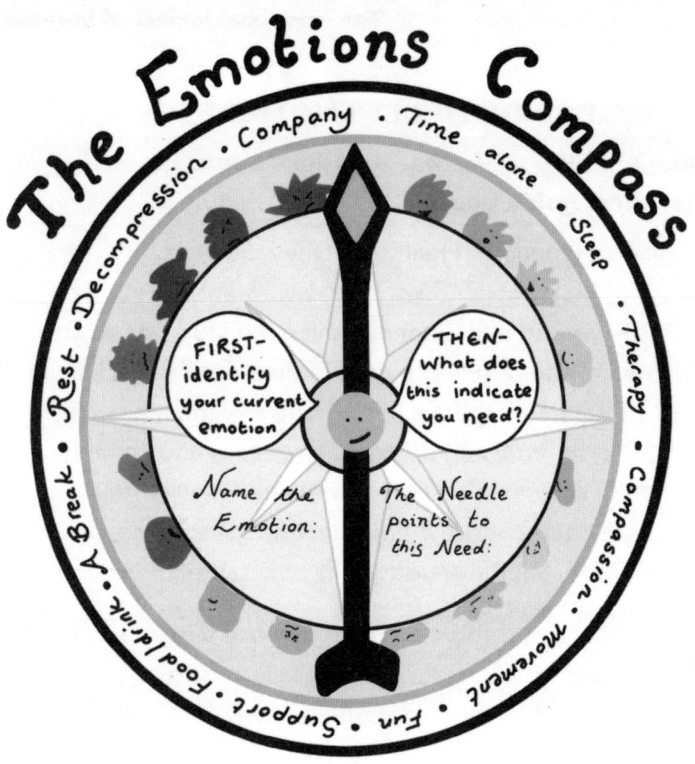

Anti-burnout Exercise 22:
The emotions compass: using difficult emotions to navigate

Think about what you are feeling. What is this emotion indicating that you need? What do you need to do to respond helpfully to this emotion and navigate through it? Are you doing anything in response to your difficult emotions that makes you feel worse and sets you off-course? There are some ideas in the compass but feel free to add your own. This exercise is about noticing how you feel and using this as an indicator for how to respond helpfully, so you can navigate through your difficult emotions.

Anti-burnout takeaways

- Many people will arrive at burnout at some point in their life. It's a common experience and not an indicator of your worth or failures.
- Burnout has an emotional, physical and life impact.
- It's important to recognize that burnout is a real thing – it has a physical impact on your brain and body; it is an injury from which we need to heal.
- When you are in burnout, it can feel like things will never change and nothing you do will make a difference – but there are many pathways out. You can and will recover.
- Burnout recovery can take time and needs patience.
- The pathways out of burnout are emotional, physical and life pathways. We have started by looking at seven emotional pathways out of burnout.

7 Emotional Pathways out of burnout

- Pathway 1: Legitimize your injury.
- Pathway 2: Hold on to hope.
- Pathway 3: Soften your shame.
- Pathway 4: Beware of bouncing back.
- Pathway 5: Don't be a sh*t to yourself.
- Pathway 6: Help your negative ninjas retreat.
- Pathway 7: Give your difficult emotions space and let them guide you.

Chapter 10
The physical impact of burnout

Let's look again at the arctic outpost and observe those zombies a bit more – watch them move slowly through life, stumble over their words, startle at noise, stare vacantly around them, unsure what to do, their frequent waking when asleep and their difficulty staying awake during the day. Although burnout may be caused by environmental factors and long-term stress, it creates physical changes in the body that account for the symptoms you see in these zombies. Research is still seeking to fully understand these physiological changes, which are likely to differ across people. What we can say for sure is that chronic firing of the stress response, with little reprieve, has changed these zombies' brains and bodies in one way or another. Burnout does not just exist in their minds and imaginations – if we were able to don our x-ray-vison goggles, we would see that burnout exists as physical changes to the brain and body structure, which explains the outward symptoms and behaviours.

Say 'hello' (and 'goodbye') to Shane and his buddies
I have found reading the research on the physical impact of burnout both validating ('Ah, that's why I feel that way!') and

terrifying ('Have I caused long-term damage to my body and brain?'). As I am trained in neuropsychology, I read about brain changes and associated neuropsychological symptoms with great interest. However, at the edge of my brain, Shane also spoke to me: 'Look what you've done – you shrunk your hippocampus (a brain region associated with memory) and prefrontal cortex (associated with executive functions – planning, organizing, attention). You enlarged your amygdala (associated with arousal, alertness and energy levels). You overworked your flight-and-fight system so much that it no longer accurately predicts when to operate. You shot your cortisol functioning to the point it no longer serves its multiple helpful purposes (such as maintaining energy levels and suppressing the immune system). You wreaked destruction on your immune system – instead of trying to help you heal, it's working overtime and fighting the very body that it's designed to help.'[1] Yes, the brain and body changes make it all make sense – my symptoms are a result of my changed physiology – but they also tap in to that terrible trio: Shane, the inner critic and the negative ninjas.

The brain and body on burnout

While Shane highlights all the harm I have caused, the negative ninjas turn to the potential catastrophic long-term impacts: the research says that people with burnout suffer more health problems, die younger, age faster.[2] Clearly my future is going to be a disaster! As the negative ninjas advance, my inner critic grabs its loudspeaker and says, 'Look what YOU have done, YOU have ruined your future!', and Shane whispers louder, 'What's wrong with you?' In my attempts to make it make sense, I've inadvertently fuelled this doom-mongering trio.

As I researched for this book, the trio popped back up, but they no longer stay so long. Yes, burnout has detrimental effects on our brain and body – that's why we feel and function the way we do, as zombies. However, we can use this knowledge to support and empower, rather than berate. Using this knowledge wisely can help us understand how we function and feel: we are not lazy, we are not underperforming, we are having to work with the effect of a burned-out brain and body. It's not our fault we got here; it's a complex mix of multiple factors, many of which were impossible to control. So, lighten the burden on yourself, throw self-blame or regret away and use this knowledge beneficially. Reading this through the lens of shame and regret isn't helpful, but releasing yourself from this burden frees up your brain and body to start getting better.

IT'S NOT ALL DOOM AND GLOOM!

Back to that research pile sitting next to me, because it's not all bad news in there. The research is still very much in its infancy – there are mixed and contradictory results about how burnout affects us physically, and it's not always clear if this is cause or effect.[3] There is a physical impact, but we can't pinpoint for sure what exactly is occurring in each brain or body for a particular person, or the extent of it. We also know that the body and brain have a remarkable ability to change: the cognitive deficits that occur in many illnesses appear to reverse as we recover, and research suggests this is also the case in burnout.[4] As I have recovered, my attention, memory, creativity and ability to plan and organize have returned (if they hadn't, I couldn't have written this book), and if we donned our x-ray goggles, we would see that this likely correlates with changes in the brain.

You can get stuck in regret and shame, which just hurts your brain even more. Or you can use your energy to understand and start to take tiny steps on the pathways out, which will help your brain and body to replenish, restrengthen, rebuild, regrow and recover. It will take time, this is not an immediate process, and you shouldn't expect it to be. It is often a zigzagged process that takes two steps forward then one back. Finally, you don't have to do it alone, other brains can and will support you through this process. Some of the cognitive and emotional impact of burnout, such as difficulty with decision making, means it can be helpful to utilize other brains as part of the recovery process, particularly to support those first steps down the pathways. Building back your brain and body is possible: you can recover, but you need to give yourself the time, space, patience and strength to do so.

7 Physical Pathways out of burnout

Physical Pathway 1: Creating space for recovery

Burnout naturally reduces your life, but it usually occurs by default rather than an intentional act. Whatever tiredness stops you doing gets ditched; you reduce activities that might make you feel good because you don't have the energy; you withdraw because things feel overwhelming. Cutting back is not the same, it is about intentionally creating a space to recover, and how it looks for you may be different for the next person. My dream was a year off, and while for some people this might be possible, for many (me included), it isn't, for practical and/or financial reasons. But if it is possible for you and works for you, then this is something to celebrate. In her book *A Year of Nothing*[5] author Emma Gannon writes about how she made this work for her. To regenerate we need space and, if possible, distance from the things that are creating stress and add weight to our branches, to allow our tree to regain energy so it can start to regrow.

Cutting back and creating space can be many different things, and we can be creative in how we do it. The extent to which you need to cut back can depend on where you are on the burnout scale (see page 33). Despite having recently started a new role, I managed to take some time off, some paid, some unpaid, that gave me time to look after myself while freeing up how I used the energy I did have, so it wasn't all directed at working. I also delayed or cut back various other roles I had, such as writing a book, which just couldn't happen. I set an 'out of office' on my email to manage expectations, didn't take on any new work (I had a standard email to say I had no capacity), stopped posting on social media and removed all social media and email apps from my phone.

Zoe, who we met in Chapter 9, stopped taking on extra shifts and managed to change her role slightly so she could work shorter, more manageable shifts and agreed flexible working so she could work a term-time-only contract. She also paused a voluntary role she was undertaking at her kids' school and decided that she would hire a cleaner once every two weeks. Zac referred himself to his company's occupational health service and, at their advice, took a period of sick leave. Once he completed a phased return, he booked regular days off over the next few months so he wasn't working a full week. He arranged to work from home part-time to reduce his commute and agreed flexi-hours so he could take additional regular days off.

The physical impact of burnout

There is no right or wrong way to cut back and create space. For some people, this may be stopping entirely, taking time off or even quitting a role. For others, it might be about restructuring their role, reducing demands or not taking on extra work. And it's not just about work, of course; it can also be about what we do to ease pressure in our roles – paying people do to tasks if we can, asking for help, accepting support, lowering our expectations, reducing demands and simplifying tasks, allowing downtime and giving ourselves permission to switch off. It's about lightening our load to enable our tree to regenerate. We need to create space and time to make sense of what's happened to us, so we can figure out the correct pathways forward. In the previous chapter, I shared some ideas for how to understand and validate your experiences, and there are a range of resources in Further Reading on page 306.

There can be practical, psychological and cognitive barriers to creating space. Practically, there may be financial or career implications. Psychologically, we can worry about how we will be perceived, be afraid of the impact of saying no, or be worried we will be left behind or that we're no longer of value. We may have to tackle some of our long-held beliefs about coping/illness/taking time off/looking after ourselves that stop us doing this (see Chapter 4), and we may need support to tackle these barriers from friends, colleagues, family or professionals. The cognitive impact may mean we have difficulty choosing between options, being able to problem solve, making decisions or even actioning them because of fatigue. This is when the use of someone's non-burned-out brain can be particularly helpful, to facilitate or action these decisions. Identifying solutions to your own personal barriers to creating space can help you circumnavigate them.

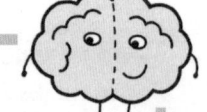

Brian the Brain reflections

- Is there anything you can step back from, reduce or pause?
- What support do you need in order to step back or pause (e.g. advice from a medical professional/referral to occupational health/discussion with your manager)?
- Do any of your beliefs create barriers to creating space?
- What are the practical barriers to creating space?
- What can you do to overcome these barriers?
- Who can you speak to help make sense of your experiences?

Physical Pathway 2: Bringing your body budget out of debt

Remember your body budget from Chapter 5? (If not, it's worth rereading that section before starting along this pathway.) Staying healthy is about keeping your body budget in balance. If it gets depleted, you need to top it up. If you have reached burnout, then your body budget is in debt – in fact, it's bankrupt. Getting it back to a healthier state is a critical part of burnout recovery. Quick top-ups won't work. Your brain and body are already affected, and there is no quick fix: it's going to take time and effort to return them to a healthy balance. The only way to return your body budget into the standard healthy budgeting zone is a long-term pattern of investment, where deposits are greater than withdrawals. You also won't have the capacity to make big changes, so any investments will have to be small and incremental. Like cash, they will grow over time, compounding slowly to have a larger effect.

The physical impact of burnout

Making deposits is about investing in looking after your body and mind. But this is not just about self-care (although it is critical): it's as much about community care, finding people and spaces that make you feel safe and supported. You don't have to do this all alone, we are all critical in creating deposits for other people, and other people can make powerful deposits to your body budget, if you let them.

Before you even start making deposits, you might have to challenge some barriers to going down this pathway. These might include beliefs about looking after yourself, asking for help and allowing yourself to rest. Everybody who hits burnout has a chronically overdrawn body budget. However, many people who have become burned out are used to putting their own needs last, have tried to be as independent as possible and have difficulty asking for help. This means they have experienced a long-term habitual norm of greater withdrawals than deposits and body-budget depletion. As a result, shifting this pattern in the opposite direction can feel weird and requires significant behavioural and belief shifts. Not only do these long-term beliefs and habitual norms get in the way of making body-budget investments, they can also stop you gaining maximum benefit from them. For example, if you have managed to rest but keep on berating yourself for taking some downtime, then this will not create the deposit in your body budget that it should.

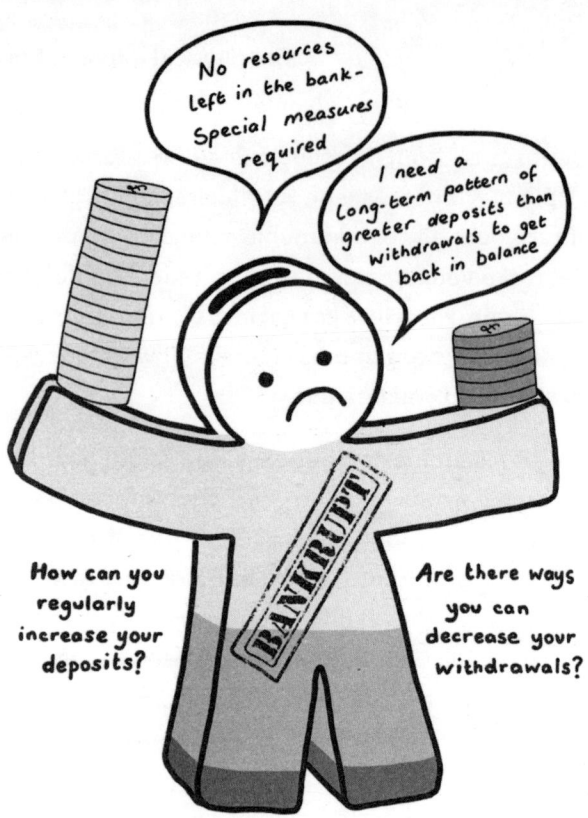

Anti-burnout Exercise 23:
Investing in your body budget: daily deposits and withdrawal tallies

Use the illustartion to think about what you can do to ensure ensure that deposits outweigh withdrawals. Moving your body out of the bankrupt zone requires regular investments, i.e. you need to regularly make more deposits than withdrawals. Take stock regularly and keep a tally if you can to ensure you are making investments. Increase your deposits as much as possible and reduce your withdrawals. There will always be withdrawals that occur which are out of your control, but it's important to try and minimize the ones you can control.

Physical Pathway 3: Working with, not against, low power mode

Your brain is a power-hungry organ. Everything it does uses energy, and some areas require more energy, so functioning declines when you have less energy to use. Your executive brain (traditionally linked to the prefrontal cortex, but like all brain functions this operates through a complex brain network) requires a lot of energy. This means it is particularly sensitive to decline when you are tired or have low energy. Executive functioning is the manager of the brain, coordinating your life (see the image below to see the tasks it is responsible for). Anyone who has ever experienced a lack of sleep (i.e. everyone) will have observed the effect of low energy on their executive function: we are more irritable and emotions hit harder; it's more difficult to stay on-task, to switch off noise, to initiate activities (especially novel ones) or to stop yourself falling into unhelpful habits. This is also the cognitive pattern we see in long-term depleted zombie brains.

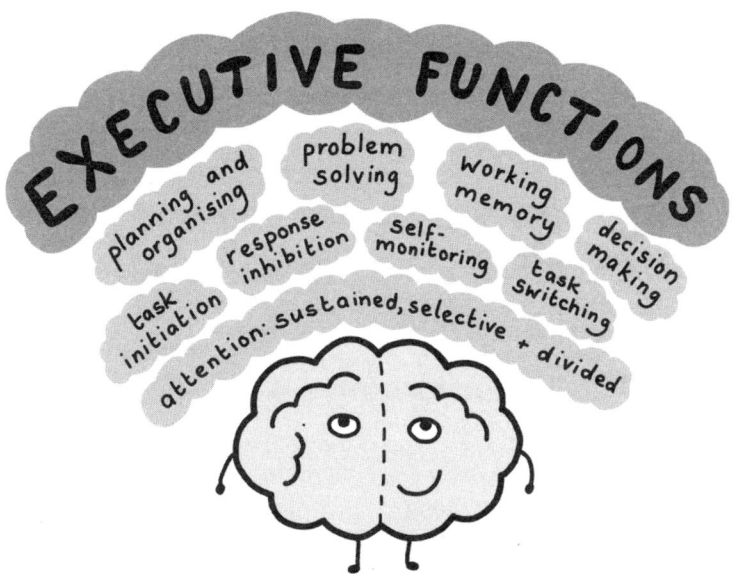

Burnout impacts cognition in multiple ways,[6] particularly executive functioning, including attention and working memory (holding information in mind).[7] This can help us understand changes in our functioning when we are burned out. Zoe told me she frequently lost track of what was doing and that she used to be decisive but now felt overwhelmed by small choices. Zac told me became distracted and irritable with background noise, and struggled to initiate new tasks, instead falling into checking his phone. I personally found myself becoming overwhelmed when there was too much going on – the radio, children talking, cooking, chatting to my husband – which overloaded my brain to the point I couldn't think or focus. All these tasks require aspects of executive functioning, which is harder for our brain when in a burned-out zombie state.

'Low power mode' is a term coined by neurologist Dr Faye Begeti in her book *The Phone Fix*[8] (which I highly recommend if your tech use is one of the stressors in your burnout tree), which I personally find helpful to describe the effects of burnout on brain functioning. She uses it to describe how the brain functions when it is depleted: like a phone entering low power mode to save battery, which conserves resources by downshifting performance. Dr Begeti states:

The executive steps down and our executive functioning deteriorates. Your brain also delegates more control to the autopilot, which defaults to short-term rewards and energy conservation.

The physical impact of burnout

This explains much of the behaviour we see in burnout, why we start to find certain tasks difficult and why we can fall into habits that aren't good for us. Low power mode is normally a temporary state until we recharge; however, this can become more of a constant state in burnout due to our chronically overdrawn body budget. This means that our functioning can change, and tasks we might have found simple before become much more difficult. We need to learn to work with our brain in low power mode because only by working with it, not against it, can we start finding the pathways out.

Working against low power mode means we try to operate like we did before, pushing through and berating and blame ourselves when things don't work. This amplifies shame as think we lack characteristics such as willpower, commitment, decisiveness and staying power when we are actually just seeing the cognitive impact of burnout. Working *with* it is about understanding the impact of burnout on our cognition, putting strategies in place to make things work as best as we can, and recognizing this occurs because of the impact of burnout rather than some major internal personal failure. Instead of saying, 'I am not good enough' or 'I have low willpower,' we shift to say, 'My cognition, particularly my executive functioning, has been impacted by burnout' or simply, 'My brain is in low power mode.' We start to locate the problem correctly, identifying the true cause and taking steps to work with it effectively.

Anti-burnout Exercise 24: Working with low power mode

The first step here is recognizing which tasks you find difficult, thinking about why this may be the case and then taking steps to make them easier. You might not always be able to pinpoint exactly *why* these tasks are difficult (e.g. the specific cognitive skills affected), but even just recognizing this occurs because your brain is in low power mode helps you understand it more and come up with solutions.

Many of the steps will be about environmental changes rather than you having to do something different, which are far easier and less energy-consuming for your brain.

This is about reducing cognitive load (and self-blame) as much as possible, so your brain has to do less work. I have included some examples from ex-zombies Zoe and Zac.

Zoe's example
- **Task I am now finding difficult:** Making decisions, e.g. what to wear in morning, what to buy in shops. More difficult when more pressure and other things going on at same time.
- **Why am I finding this difficult?** Difficulties with executive functioning as brain is in low power mode.
- **What can I do to make this easier?** Make decisions when less pressure, e.g. choose clothes the night before, make shopping list before going to the shop.

Zac's example
- **Task I am now finding difficult:** Being distracted at work when it's noisy. Becoming irritable.
- **Why am I finding this difficult?** Difficulties with attention and tuning out background noise. Reduced capacity to deal with stressors.
- **What can I do to make this easier?** Do simpler task in office and more complex tasks at home. Wear noise-cancelling headphones. Move to meeting room when need to, to keep attention on task.

Physical Pathway 4: Shifting your expectations

Okay, you've cut back, you've upped your body budget investments and you're working with low power mode. Fantastic, you have set yourself down a helpful pathway out of burnout. Now we need to look at what you do on a daily basis. Because if you are anything like me, even though you know logically that your brain is not functioning how it normally does, it will continue to make judgements based on your pre-burnout capacity rather than on how it functions now. Let me explain. When in burnout, I absolutely knew theoretically that my brain wasn't functioning on tip-top form and that my body was under par. But did my brain take this into account in my daily predictions of what I could do? Ha ha, of course it didn't!

The brain constantly uses past experiences to make predictions for the future, and this includes estimates of how much we think we will get done and how long things will take us. During burnout, I continued to make these estimates based on pre-burnout functioning – setting myself up to fail all over the place. I would dictate that letter in about an hour (realistic estimate based on pre-zombie Emma), but it would take me three hours. I could respond to all my emails first thing in the morning in about twenty minutes, but it took me all morning. I could cook the meal in about half an hour, but thirty minutes later I was still debating how to start. Low power mode and fatigue meant that everything was more difficult and took longer, but my predictions didn't allow for this. This just added more stress to my burnout tree: I kept on trying to achieve the impossible, working longer and harder to complete what I planned to do and rushing things (which is stressful), and it fed into feeling I was failing (because I never made my unrealistic predicted targets) and letting people down.

A major shift that started me down a pathway out of burnout was to alter my expectation so that my predictions of what I could do, and how long things would take me, became (at least a bit more) realistic. This alleviated the pressure in multiple ways – I did less, had more time to do tasks, no longer tried to achieve things in unrealistic time periods and rushed less. It also opened unexpected pockets of time that gave me some space. Instead of creating greater stress and withdrawals from my body budget, I was instead using that time to create greater deposits.

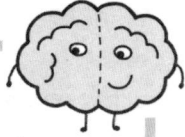

Brian the Brain reflections

- Think about what expectations you need to shift to make your life more manageable. These can be expectations about what you can achieve, how long tasks will take or how much you can do in a day.
- How can you shift these expectations, so they are more realistic?

The physical impact of burnout

Physical Pathway 5: Working with minimal capacity

Your capacity is significantly reduced in burnout due to reduced brain functioning and energy levels – your capacity cup has gone from a chunky soup mug to a thimble-sized doll's cup. It can carry much less, and although hopefully you've already cut back demands (see page 220), ongoing demands are just an inevitable part of most people's lives, particularly (as we've seen in Chapter 7) if you are a parent or carer. However, if your cup has shrunk to a thimble then it's often not just full, it's teetering above the brim, a vulnerable meniscus (that strange convex brim above a cup) just waiting for a tiny thing to burst it. This means two things:

1. You need to be very careful and conscious about what you let into your cup (when possible).

2. You need to regularly take extra steps to increase your capacity, because doing so, even just a bit, makes your cup less likely to overflow. This might include taking a short break by doing something brief that relaxes you (for me it's stepping into my garden for a few minutes).

The irony, though, is that when we are at full capacity, the very things that increase our capacity can feel like they are too much effort, and they tend to fall to the wayside. But even teeny-tiny expansions are worthwhile, as these little moments help our cup expand slightly. You may want to refer back to the exercises at the end of Chapter 7 to think about ways you can increase your capacity, even just a little bit.

Physical Pathway 6: Capacity overflow and overwhelm

As your shrunken capacity cup is now tiny, and therefore almost always full, you are never far away from overwhelm, or what I call Creamola-foam* cup (I am a child of the 1980s after all) – and it only takes a tiny thing to get there (see page 220). Overwhelm occurs when your capacity overflows – you don't have brain space to deal with what's going on, your brain cannot cope with the information coming at it, your cognition goes haywire and you can't see a way forward. Your body goes into high flight-and-fight zone – you might panic, feel totally lost or freeze. We all experience this sometimes; if we have lots of capacity it is usually the big life events that get us there. However, when you are burned out, it can be the tiniest things that gets you there – one little seemingly innocent comment, a minor problem, a call from the school, a forgotten key ingredient for the evening meal (yes, I did cry over a lack of tinned tomatoes) … Bam, wham, kerplunk! You have no capacity left and it Creamola-foams* your brain into a bubbling, steaming, overflowing mess.

Learning to deal with overwhelm is critical for burnout, because these tiny innocuous incidents that overflow our thimble-sized cups can be major blocks on the paths out. An overwhelmed brain gets stuck and reverts to its bad old ways. The terrible trio of shame, inner critic and negative ninjas see a chink through which they can enter. The seemingly tiny barrier gathers momentum to become an Indiana Jones-style rolling boulder that pushes you back down the path, or worse still, knocks you flat and you have to rebuild again. By learning to deal with overwhelm when it happens, because it will, you can stop this tiny thing gathering momentum to become a giant boulder in your path.

---

* This was a drink made from adding water to Creamola foam powder, which bubbled and fizzed up and always spilt over the cup.

The physical impact of burnout

Anti-burnout Exercise 25: Six steps to stop the overwhelm rolling stone

1. STOP
Recognize you are overwhelmed. What are your indicators? (Mine are feeling frozen and not knowing what to do.)

2. STEP AWAY
If you can, step away from what is making you feel overwhelmed into a calming space, e.g. if you are at your computer go for a brief walk. Even just a moment in a different space can help calm you.

3. SLOW THE SYMPTOMS
Breathing exercises can be helpful here. Other ways to slow the symptoms include movement, grounding exercises, music, closing your eyes – anything that helps calm your body down.

4. SKEDDADLE IT OUT OF YOUR BRAIN
It can be helpful for some people to do this straight away, but other people might prefer to wait – do what works best for you. Get everything that's causing overwhelm out of your brain and onto paper so you can make sense of it. I call this a brain dump: draw a brain outline on a sheet of paper and write or draw everything that's making you feel overwhelmed.

5. SHARE THE SCARIES
If you have a safe and compassionate person around then utilize their brain. We know overwhelm and burnout

effects brain functioning, so having another brain to help sort out overwhelm casts a more objective eye over what's going on. It's always helpful to have an extra 86 billion neurons working on something, for the additional problem solving it can bring.

6. SORT IT OUT

This step is about recognizing what you need to do about the things causing overwhelm. I find it helpful to sort things into three categories:

1. **Immediate first steps:** Easy things you or other people can do now.
2. **Longer-term plans:** These can make things feel more in control. They could be things that need no action now so can just sit on the side-burner, or longer-term actions that are needed in the next few days/weeks, so you can disregard them in the moment.
3. **Throw them away:** Consider the things you can disregard and don't need to worry about. You may need to take some immediate steps (e.g. an email response to say no to something) before you can throw things in this pile.

BONUS 7th STEP: STOPPING FUTURE ROLLING STONES

You may want to think about things you can do to reduce overwhelm reoccurring. Use the capacity cup exercise on page 47. You could also use strategies around saying no and self-preservation in the next chapter.

Physical Pathway 7: Protecting and managing your energy

Taylor Swift is here to introduce this pathway with something she said while I was writing this book:

Think of your energy as if it's expensive, as if it's like a luxury item. Not everyone can afford it ... What you spend your energy on, that's the day.

How are you using your energy? Before burnout you probably never really had to think about this. Your energy supply wasn't limited but it was abundant, and when it got low, you were able to top it up again with sleep or rest. You were like a relatively new phone, with a well-functioning battery. Now your energy reserves are more like an older phone – you have much less energy, the battery depletes quicker and it's much more difficult to recharge. You don't have abundant energy for keeping multiple needless apps all on the go at once, using up all your charge; you need to prioritize how you use your energy. Use too much, and it's not a case of a quick top-up; it can create an energy hangover that lasts for days. One of the ways we do this is we fall into a boom-and-bust cycle: when we feel good, we use loads of energy, which then depletes us for several days in a row.

Now, your energy is a precious resource: you have to carefully consider how you use it and make conscious intentional decisions about where to invest it, in a way that's meaningful to you. There are many different models and techniques for managing energy that I have used clinically. Low energy is common in many medical conditions, such as after a brain injury, where fatigue is one of the most common symptoms. One that tends to resonate with people is Christine Miserandino's spoon theory,[9] which she used to explain living with her condition lupus but which is now used in many conditions where you have to consider energy use. Here's how spoon theory works:

1. Everybody starts with a certain number of spoons of energy per day – for many (particularly young and well) this is unlimited, but burnout will have affected how many spoons you have. How many spoons do you start the day with? Let's imagine you start with 12 with burnout. (It will take a bit of experimenting to find how many energy spoons you normally start with.)

2. Do you need to subtract any? Some things might mean you need to detract spoons immediately – for example, a bad night's sleep (subtract 1) and a cold (subtract another).

3. What do you need to do today? Everything takes up spoons, some may take up more spoons than others. For example, small things may use 1 spoon: getting dressed or reading a book. Other things use a greater number of spoons: cooking a meal may take 3 spoons; going to the gym or meeting a friend may take 5.

4. Once you have used all your spoons, that is your energy used for today. You can borrow from tomorrow to do more things, but you must recognize that you will then start with fewer spoons of energy tomorrow.

This isn't an exact science; we are estimating how many spoons of energy we have to start the day and how many spoons each task uses. This normally becomes clearer once you've tried the

The physical impact of burnout

exercise a few times. However, it's a visual way to actively think about your energy use, how to use this in a meaningful way and how to balance energy use with what you need to do. As you recover from burnout, the number of spoons you have each day is likely to increase, so you can revisit this exercise to adapt it as you move out of burnout. Let's make this work for you:

> **Anti-burnout Exercise 26:**
> **Managing your energy spoons**
>
> How many spoons do you have at the start of the day?
>
> Do you need to detract any (for example, due to illness, lack of sleep)?
>
> How many spoons do activities take? Write your normal activities here and how many spoons they take. When you do a new activity, add it in. Remember these are estimates.
>
> How will you use your spoons today?
>
> How many spoons are you left with at the end of the day? If you are left with a negative number, you will have to subtract this from tomorrow's spoons.

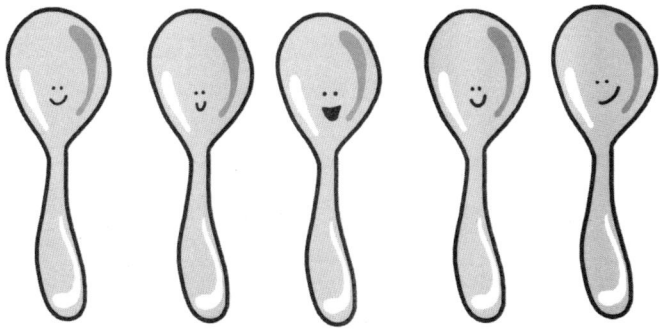

Anti-burnout takeaways

- Burnout has a physical impact on your brain and body.
- We can consider burnout an injury that you need to recover from, and that takes time and is a gradual process.
- Understanding the physical impact of burnout can help you understand your symptoms.
- Reading about the physical symptoms of burnout can be scary and may be a trigger that lets shame in. It's important to find ways to manage this.
- Your body can heal from the physical impact of burnout.

7 Physical Pathways out of burnout

- Pathway 1: Cut back to recover.
- Pathway 2: Bring your body budget out of debt.
- Pathway 3: Work with low power mode.
- Pathway 4: Shift your expectations.
- Pathway 5: Work with significantly reduced capacity.
- Pathway 6: Manage capacity overflow and overwhelm.
- Pathway 7: Protect and intentionally manage your energy.

Chapter 11
Piecing your life back together after burnout

Burnout impacts us emotionally and physically, but the fallout this has on our life is pervasive. Exhaustion shrinks our world: it stops us partaking in joy; it builds up tasks into impossible mountains; it takes control from us. Shame makes us shrink from those who help us grow; makes us feel like a burden and hide our humanity from the world. Our inner critic questions our value and makes us believe that we don't have a place in the world. Burnout shatters our lives and breaks the very core of who we are into tiny pieces.

What I call the 'life impact' of burnout is all the things that it has stopped us doing or has made us start doing. It is the collateral damage – the parts that become neglected and the meaning we lose as result. It is the friendships we can no longer nurture because we have no energy or that we avoid for fear of being a burden or exposing our shame. It is the loss of the activities we enjoyed, which fall to the wayside because they no longer bring joy or partaking in them requires too much effort or resources. It is the habits we fall into, that we know perpetuate the cycle but from which we can't break free. It is the metaphorical and literal mountains that build up into unsurmountable tasks indicative of our failures: the emails not responded to, the paperwork piles falling off the sideboard, the mountains of mess that gather around the house. It is the loss of control as we no longer feel we are even loosely holding the strings of life together. It is the shattering of our identity as the pieces that made us break away, leaving us questioning who we are. Piecing your life back together is about both building back the parts of your life you want and leaving those behind that you don't. Some of these parts you might want to leave behind, but some you may grieve for – parts of you that you have lost or a part of life in which you can no longer partake. You may also grieve for future anticipated life paths that you no longer believe are possible.

The impact of burnout on my life

As I fell into burnout, layers of my life stripped away, leaving the unrecognizable burned-out Emma zombie. Socializing felt too much, as I had lost all fun, ideas and sometimes (at peak exhaustion) even the ability to follow a conversation. I withdrew, as I knew I would be rubbish company anyway. Shame stopped me from telling people how I felt, then berated me because I hadn't told them. Basic nurturing activities, which had helped me through tough times before, slipped away and were replaced with staring vacantly into my phone while shoving beige frozen goods into the oven, where I found Shane staring at back me. Activities that previously gave me joy became chores to get through. With creativity a long-lost memory, I no longer felt the urge to express myself and capture my ideas through reading, writing and drawing – activities that were an integral part of me. Unsent invoices and unanswered emails became insurmountable Everests in my mind. Like me, my life felt like an unmanageable mess. I had lost control over significant parts and failed to get joy or purpose out of those that remained. Each loss shrunk my life and broke further pieces from me, so that I left a trail of myself behind me everywhere I went.

STORIES FROM THE ZOMBIE ARMY

The ex-zombies told me similar stories. Zoe stopped nearly everything outside of work. Her friends gradually stopped texting as she never replied. She felt she had lost connection with her partner as she was too tired to have proper catch-ups once the kids were in bed, like they used to. Her nightly wine that started during the Covid pandemic became two or three to help her sleep. It stopped her mind racing, but she felt more exhausted the next morning. Her house was no longer a relaxing place: it was messy and out of control and she felt unable to do anything about it. This fuelled her inner critic, which told her that everyone else was managing and she was useless.

Zac told me he felt he had lost control of his finances and was regularly behind with paying bills and was getting charged for this. He no longer looked after his diet like he used to and couldn't face cooking so he relied on ready meals and takeaways (he jokingly told me his closest friend was the delivery driver). He didn't want to go to the gym, which was previously his main social network outside of work, as he didn't want people to see how far he 'had slipped backwards' or his 'lack of resilience, drive and motivation', stating that he was weak-willed and the kind of person he had previously judged harshly.

What do all zombies have in common?

When we look at our zombies, we can see some patterns: most of them in the arctic outpost have withdrawn from social contact, stopped doing activities they enjoy and feel like they are falling behind with the tasks of life or just life itself. Nearly all our zombies fell into some unhelpful habits that might be self-soothing short term but that make them more zombie-like in the long term. If you'd looked out as they entered the outpost, you'd have noticed a trail of cast-off parts of their identity as far as the eye can see, which they have gradually lost to reach the zombie stage. They are shadows of their former selves; in fact, many of them don't even know who they are anymore. I have seen similar patterns with nearly everybody with burnout I have worked with – the commonality in how burnout impacts on life is striking. It ruptures your life path and shrinks your life. Everyone is wondering how they will ever get out, because no matter which way they turn, the paths that reconnect them to their lives seem mountainous and require more energy than they can muster.

Getting out of the arctic outpost

We've already seen there are many pathways out of burnout, and the more steps we take down these seemingly treacherous overgrown pathways, the more they become smooth, paved paths that are easier to find and walk along. And the more paths we go down, the more they merge, opening up to become tracks, roads and highways, then perhaps even super-highways, that guide us out more easily. However, some of the pathways are initially harder to go down than others.

Piecing your life back together after burnout

Many of the pathways out so far have involved looking inwards and supporting yourself, but that is not enough. To reach the super-highways, we must follow paths that help us look outwards and regrow our connections with the world. However, at the start, these paths can feel like the most overgrown, scary and insurmountable to go down. They have complex barriers in their way that we need to overcome – shame, doubt, outdated beliefs, habitual patterns, societal norms and expectations, our own shoulds and musts. These hurdles make us question whether we would be better to turn back to the relative safety of arctic isolation. Going down these pathways often requires work before we start to reintegrate with the world – to tackle our inner taboos and beliefs, to soften our shame and to be gentle and compassionate with ourselves (see Chapter 4) when we misstep or go backwards (because we will). It requires small fairy-steps forward, alongside belief that following this path WILL build something much better.

As we take these teeny-tiny steps forward, we are not retracing our steps that got us here; we are finding new ways forward that will enable us to get to a different place. A place in which it is worth staying. A place that will let our tree regenerate and regrow. A place that will not just push us back into burnout again. A place where we can thrive. You do not have exit the same way that you got here – another way out is possible.

These pathways out of burnout are low energy to start with. For when we are burned out, we do not have the cognitive or energy reserves for big decisions or big actions. These can come later. Let's start small.

7 Life Pathways out of burnout

Life Pathway 1: No longer quashing what you want and need

Burnout commonly results from quashing your needs and wants. This can become long-term patterns: we need to please others to feel worthwhile or put our own needs last because we don't think we are worth looking after. Recovering from burnout is about shifting this to really start to understand your needs and what you want so you can build a life around them, rather than ignoring them. This quote from the podcast *Illuminated: In Pieces* by Hana Walker-Brown[1] really stuck with me during my own burnout:

Burnout is an invitation to stop and think. To create what you want out of the pieces of your life.

To do this, you need to think about what you want and need. What YOU want and need, not what other people or society tell you that you should want and need. By understanding this, you can set the direction of your path rather than just pushing forward in any which way that happens to open up and pull you towards it. Once you know where you want to head, you can start to see which teeny-tiny steps to take. You can also recognize missteps, or when you fall into old habits (taking on more, being busy all the time), which seem like you are finding your way out but are actually circular paths that will eventually lead us back to the burnout arctic outpost.

When ex-zombie Zoe looked at this, she decided she wanted a job that would enable her to be comfortable enough financially and spend time with her children. She wanted to reconnect with her husband and enjoy time with her wider family and friends. She wanted to feel appreciated at work and did not want to go for promotions (as she was being pushed into it). Ex-zombie Zac told me he wanted to feel like he had some time and to be able to go at a slower pace. He wanted to ensure his work life didn't regularly detract from his personal life. He wanted to reconnect with hobbies he had lost, such as basketball, and to look after his health. By identifying simply what they wanted, Zoe and Zac could make sure their steps forwards were consistent with what they wanted.

Now this may seem like a ridiculously simple exercise, but for many of us it has hidden layers of complexity. We may have subjugated our needs for so long that we no longer know what we need, let alone want. Remember, you are thinking about what you want, not what you think you SHOULD want or what other people want for you. Yes, of course other people's needs are important, but so are yours. And sometimes deciding what you don't want can be the first step to figuring out what you DO want.

Some reflections before we start:

- What is important to you?
- What energizes you (normally, when you are not burned out)?
- When do you feel most content/happy/satisfied?
- What makes you unhappy/dissatisfied?
- If you were to look back on your life at the age of 100, what would you want to see?
- What do you not want any longer (this is sometimes easier to start with)? What would you like to see/do instead?

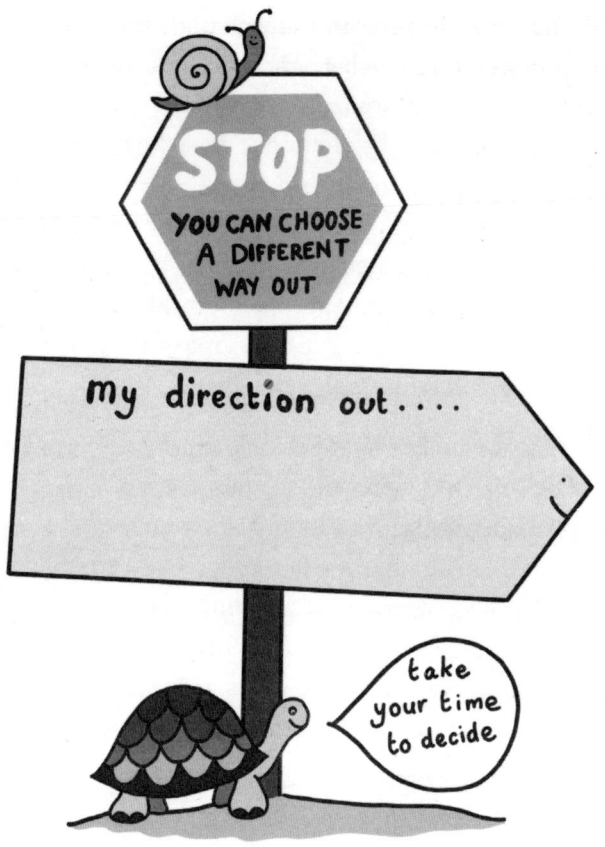

Anti-burnout Exercise 27:
Signposting the direction out of burnout

Fill in the signpost with what you want. This might take time to work out, and things may pop into your head at random points. This is also never a finished exercise, so come back to it regularly and reconsider. All you are doing at the moment is pointing yourself in the direction of 'out', towards a life that works for you.

Life Pathway 2: Rebuilding your identity – putting some jigsaw pieces of yourself back together

Who are you? What makes you, you? Burnout can rupture our identity and leave the pieces of ourselves strewn on the floor like a broken-up jigsaw puzzle at our feet. But it can also bring into question which parts of our identity were built on shaky foundations. These pieces are also on the floor at our feet, but we no longer want them to be part of our identity. It can be tempting to grasp at these puzzle pieces again and slot them in, because they have been part of us for so long, but leaving them behind creates new spaces in your identity, which you can then fill with who you really are, something meaningful to you.

But that's all longer term (and for the next chapter). Right now, we are just starting to rebuild and deciding which pieces we will choose to intentionally leave behind. This is just the first step in putting the pieces of yourself back together – like with a jigsaw puzzle, we start with the edges or a prominent part and then we build the more complex parts up over time. You also get to choose which parts you thought were an important part of your identity but were actually things you thought you should do, that other people believed were right for you, that society subscribed you to. In reality, these pieces were never meant to be part of your identity: believing they were and behaving according to them may have contributed to burnout. By leaving these behind and building a puzzle you truly believe in, and acting in accordance with it, you strengthen your tree going forward.

The Anti-Burnout Book

Anti-burnout Exercise 28:

Part 1: Rebuilding the first pieces of your identity jigsaw puzzle

Our identities are all constructed out of multiple components. They are built on what we do, what we enjoy, what we find meaningful, what we identify with, who we spend time with and where we feel safe to express our needs and be ourselves, rather than having to hide or mask who we are. This changes over time: we shed old pieces and discover more of what it means to be us throughout our lives. Don't worry too much about finding definitive answers to these questions, because this is an evolving puzzle. Fill in the important parts of you in the jigsaw puzzle and think about how you can start to reconnect to them:

- What makes you, you?
- What do you do that makes you feel like you are being true to yourself and at peace with who you are?
- When do you feel most like yourself?
- Where do you feel most at ease?

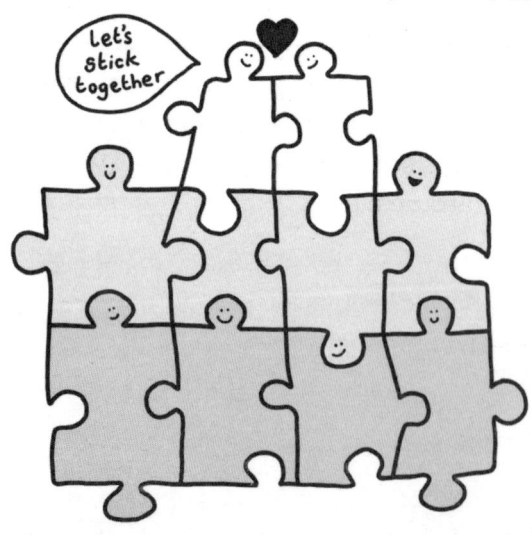

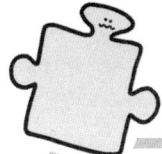
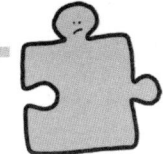

Piecing your life back together after burnout

Part 2: The pieces you are leaving behind (because they never really fitted anyway)

This is where you start to really question how you defined and valued yourself. For me, it was about ditching old ideas of success, about being busy and productive and what they meant about me. They had not served me, I did not really believe them and I didn't want them to be part of who I am. These pieces may have been fragilely holding your identity puzzle together before burnout but ultimately, they were part of your undoing, unsustainable and easy-to-shatter pieces that can make the whole puzzle more likely to crumble. Fill in the parts you will be leaving behind in the jigsaw puzzle:

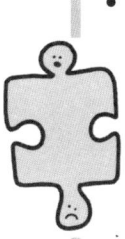

- Which pieces did burnout shatter, because they were fragile and not meant to be there?
- Which elements of your identity do you think are based on what society told you you should be?
- What shaky ground did you base your value or self-worth on? Perhaps it was productivity, your achievements or being perfect? Or maybe (like me) being a resilient, strong person who could push through and keep going? Was your identity around being the good girl (or boy) who complied and shrunk your own needs to meet those of others?
- Which pieces of your identity do you want to leave behind because they no longer define or serve you?

By ditching the pieces that are not serving you, you allow space for who you really are and to build back a more sustainable and stronger identity.

Life Pathway 3: Regrowing your roots and reconnecting with the world

Nearly every zombie I have met, and there have been many, has disconnected from their world in some way. For some it has been total withdrawal, for others their world had shrunk around them. The remaining components are normally the parts they are left with, rather than ones they have chosen. All too often, the remaining parts are the heavy stress-inducing ones, because all energy has been directed to firefight these stressors in order to reduce or control them. Ironically, the parts that fell to the wayside were the ones that truly connected us to the world, which supported us, gave us purpose and (in 'normal' times at least) made us feel good. The contraction of life as we entered the arctic tundra was an attempt to survive, but actually it just made us contract further, because it withdrew all that was meaningful from life.

It's important to emphasize that reduction and withdrawal is an important part of burnout recovery. But all too often the parts we cut are actually our roots that make us stronger rather the stressors in our branches. By intentionally cutting back rather than incidentally shrinking our life (see page 235) we create space to reconnect and grow our roots through tiny fairy-steps. There is no one right way – we can't be too prescriptive, it's not a one-size-fits-all. Initial steps can be seen as little experiments, through which you will discover what is right for you at that point. If we just take fairy-steps, it is easy to retract a step and take a different direction if we discover it is the wrong path for us at that point in time.

Piecing your life back together after burnout

Anti-burnout Exercise 29: Growing your roots through teeny-tiny fairy-steps

This exercise is about taking tiny steps to regrow your roots at a pace that is right for you. It's about reconnecting you to what matters. My fairy-steps were initially reconnecting with friends via messages, starting gradually to meet up again in real life with people who energize me. I also started reconnecting with exercise via gentle classes that felt manageable, such as yin yoga. Fill in your fairy-steps to think about how you will start regrowing your roots.

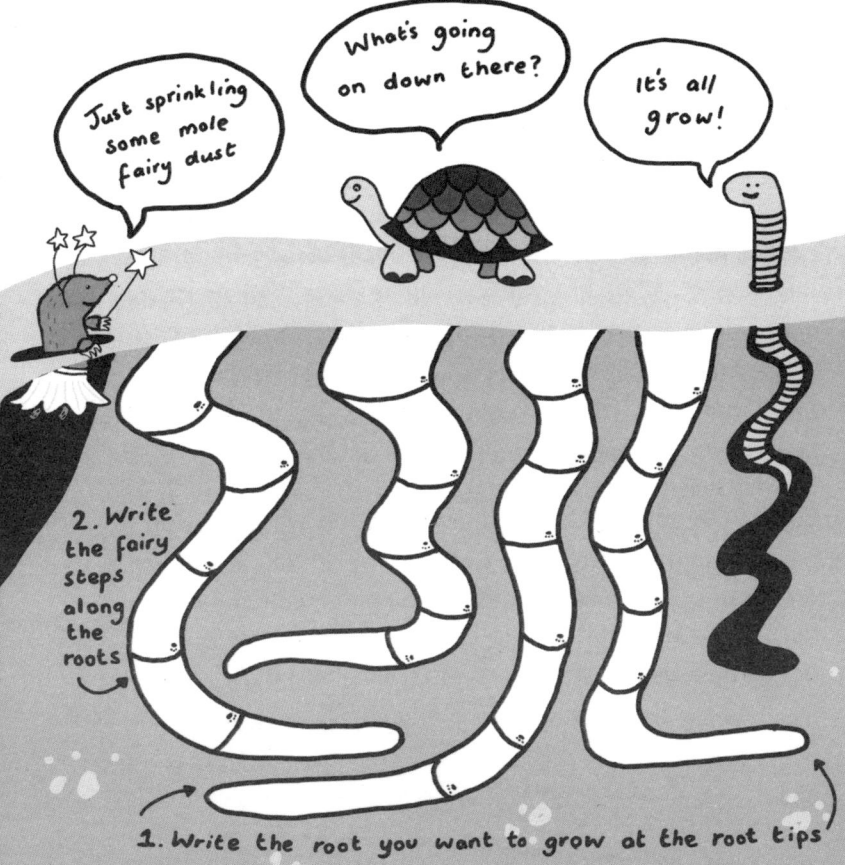

Life Pathway 4: What makes you shine? Recapturing joy, awe and wonder

Burnout knocks the joy out of us. But it's not just joy that we lose. As the negative-ninja army advances through your brain, it strategically knocked out a range of feel-good emotions: awe, wonder, amusement, fun, happiness, pleasure, anticipation, pride. The negative-ninja army has captured these emotions in a double bind: firstly, we retreat from things that made us feel good, then, ironically, the things that previously made us feel good fail to elicit these reactions (and sometimes even made us feel bad). For example, reading books had been one of the real joys in my life but became so wearisome that it just felt stressful and reminded me of all the things I could no longer do.

Feel-good emotions may seem lost to the past but they are not: we just need to recapture them from the negative-ninja army. How do we do this? By remembering what made us shine previously and doing it regardless, even though we don't want to, in small, manageable ways. This is not about jumping back in expecting joy – that's too much to expect. It's about reconnecting with things that made us shine in small, gradual ways. Although it feels like these past joys are tarnished, never to return, once we reach out, re-engage and feel even a little bit good doing them, we start to release the chains around them and reclaim those feelings we once had.

One of the ways I recaptured my feel-good emotions was taking time every day to look around my garden and notice what had grown, despite me having neglected it for a long time. I hushed my inner critic with compassion and let myself notice the flowers emerging, what had self-seeded, which birds were visiting. As the flowers grew, my feel-good emotions started to grow alongside them. Walking round my garden with a cup of tea, just looking and noticing, became part of my daily routine. This grew to become my regular morning routine and then my break routine when I was working at home, and it still is. Since then, my garden has become a major source of joy, hope and anticipation: I have never previously noticed so many flowers, birds nesting, baby birds, new growth – they have always been there, but burnout turned me towards them and they now give me more feel-good emotions than they ever have before. Think about how you will recapture joy and other feel-good emotions with the prompts below.

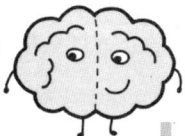

Brian the Brain reflections

- What three things used to make you shine?
- How can you reconnect with these things in a small way?

Life Pathway 5: REST IS POWER

At some point, peak burnout, after making the kids tea with nothing particular left to do, I was wandering around the kitchen in a state of unease and high alert when my husband came in, looked at me and said, 'You've forgotten how to rest.' The accuracy of this statement hit me hard. I had forgotten; my always-on brain didn't know how to rest anymore. I decided in that moment I had to relearn how to rest, to think about this as a skill that I could become better at and learn how to do again. Because rest is a skill, it's not something that just happens (particularly in burnout); it's something we have to do, plan and sometimes even fight for.

The Anti-Burnout Book

You'll have probably spotted the irony of my statement 'relearn to rest'. You may remember from previous chapters that resting was never one of my key skills, and this was certainly one of my branches that contributed to burnout. 'I rest by doing,' I used to say, and I was a master of powering through when my battery was already depleted. In reality, resting wasn't a skill I had to relearn; I had to learn it from scratch.

If this is the case for you, the first thing you have to do is to break down the large boulder that is blocking your path: your beliefs about rest. You can use the exercise opposite to help with this. Because the reality is, rest is power. Rest gives us the energy we need to survive and thrive. Rest gives us space to think, breath, reflect and challenge, and take action when needed. Poet Tricia Hersey even describes rest as resistance,[2] because it challenges the system that makes us be constantly productive as a definition of success, to the detriment of our basic needs. 'Powering on' is a misnomer – it should be called 'draining on', because continuing to do this when we need to recharge is draining us of vital resources and putting us into a chronically overdrawn body budget (and we all know what that leads to). Rest is a basic need, not something you earn, deserve or reserve for when you reach an end point or achieve something. It needs to be built into your day as a norm, not an unobtainable luxury good reserved for when you can afford to give it time. I have included some books in the Further Reading on page 306 that I found helpful to change my beliefs and learn rest as a skill that I could incorporate in my daily routine.

Anti-burnout Exercise 30: Learning to rest, like really rest

Once you've smashed that beliefs boulder about rest into smithereens and cleared the path forward, it's time to start learning to really rest. It's time to develop this as an integral skill in your life, which is about learning to rest responsively and proactively – both are important. There are three steps to this:

1. **Understanding what rest means to you:** What is restful to you will differ according to your energy levels and mood. There are several helpful models to really understand and learn to rest. For example, Dr Dalton-Smith, author of *Sacred Rest*, breaks down rest into seven different categories, as follows: physical, mental, emotional, social, sensory, creative and spiritual.[3] Suzy Reading, author of *Rest to Reset*, defines eight pillars of rest to help you determine what you need to energize you.[4]

However, in the middle of burnout we need to make it simple. List all the things that replenish your energy. These can include:

- Typical resting activities, such as napping.
- Activities that settle your mind, such as reading.
- Activities that boost your energy or put you into a flow state, such as being creative.

Now use the battery over the page to think about which activities work at different energy levels. For example, when your energy is fully depleted, something that helps you physically rest will enable you to stop and recharge.

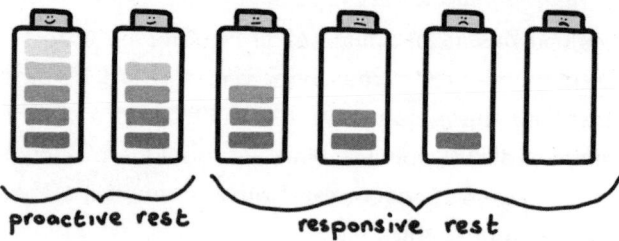

2. **Responsive rest:** Notice that your energy is draining and respond with a matched activity to address your body's needs. For example, if you feel physically tired, you might take a nap. If you notice your brain is struggling to take in information, you might take a brain break, such as walking outside. If you feel your muscles are tightening, you may do some stretches. We already know that noticing how you are feeling is a skill in itself (see Chapter 2), and it is also a skill to match those feelings with a suitable restful or re-energizing activity. These are skills you can practise, so you can learn what works for you. Use the battery to stop regularly and recognize your energy levels, label what you are feeling, then pick the activity from your list that you think will work best.
3. **Proactive rest:** Incorporate rest proactively into your day. It is not just about replenishing when depleted, it is also about keeping your energy topped up regularly even when you still have some. Proactive rest keeps you healthy and improves functioning and wellbeing. From my experience, this is what people (me included) are

worst at. They keep on going until they can do no more and are forced to rest. Proactive rest is about taking regular breaks and planning re-energizing activities as a normal part of your day, ensuring you don't work intensely for too long and understanding that your brain and body function better if they can pause. This is not always easy, because we are used to powering (er, I mean draining) through. Historically I have been a nightmare at this, but when writing this book, I really started to put this into practise – I made sure I had at least a ten-minute break for every hour I wrote. I also planned breaks between meetings and ensured I had them blocked off in my diary. Proactive rest is not just about breaks – it's also about factoring in restful and re-energizing activities as a standard part of your day, rather than just resting responsively when you need it.

Life Pathway 6: Embracing the messiness

Burnout impacts on so much of life, it can start to feel like the mess literally and metaphorically surrounds us and takes over. We are a mess, life is a mess and our house/paperwork/work/emails/other aspects of life may be a mess too. Everything feels stressful, overwhelming and out of control. In a world that reveres organization, tidiness, self-control and resilience, the terrible trio (negative ninjas, inner critic and shame) grab hold of our messy life and shout, 'What's wrong with you? Why can't you manage? You will never feel in control again!' It makes the mess about moral value: not something that has happened, but rather a fundamental reflection on us. We think that surely the path to recovery is by regaining control?

However, this quest for control can set us up in a burnout trap: if we believe we will only feel better if we are in control again, then we work, work, work, using all our energy, to regain control. All of us want to feel in control of this messy and complex world in which we live, but it's a futile use of our limited energy to try and control the uncontrollable. Instead, to find the pathway out we need to relinquish control, at least temporarily, of what we can't currently control and accept the mess.

This pathway out can feel like we are going backwards, until we realize it is guiding us out. It requires learning to live with the messiness that we have an urge to control. We can't control everything, and what we can control shifts as life's demands change. Burnout shrinks our circle of control. Relinquishing control of what's not currently within our control ironically helps us feel more in control. By learning to live with the inevitable messiness of life, we can accept this, for the moment at least. We can limit the unnecessary use of energy and instead direct this effectively towards what IS within our control and what WILL make us feel better. Burnout has made life messy in some way, and to survive we need to learn to rest and enjoy ourselves even when this is happening. During burnout, I found Oliver Burkeman's words from his book *Meditations for Mortals* helpful:

> *Our problem, it turns out, wasn't that we hadn't found the right way to achieve control over life ... Our problem was imagining any of this might be possible in the first place.*[5]

Anti-burnout Exercise 31: Learning to rest among the mess

Step 1: Recognizing that mess has no moral value

The first step is undoing the moral value you have been placing on the messy smoking embers that burnout has left. The physical or metaphorical mess has no moral value or inherent meaning. It has nothing to do with your worth or what kind of person you are. It does not define you.

- Have you been holding yourself responsible for the mess?
- Think about what meaning you have been giving the mess left behind by burnout.
- If this is unhelpful, what can you tell yourself instead?

Step 2: Relinquishing control

This is a hard one, because humans like to feel in control, some more so than others. This is not about relinquishing control over everything, it's about recognizing that we can only control so much, identifying what we can currently control and focusing our energy on this.

Use the diagram to think about:

- How has burnout shrunk your circle of control?
- Are you using your energy to try to control things that are not currently within your control (the outer circle)? How is this impacting on you?
- What can you relinquish control of (the outer circle) so you can direct your energy more beneficially to the inner circle?

The Anti-Burnout Book

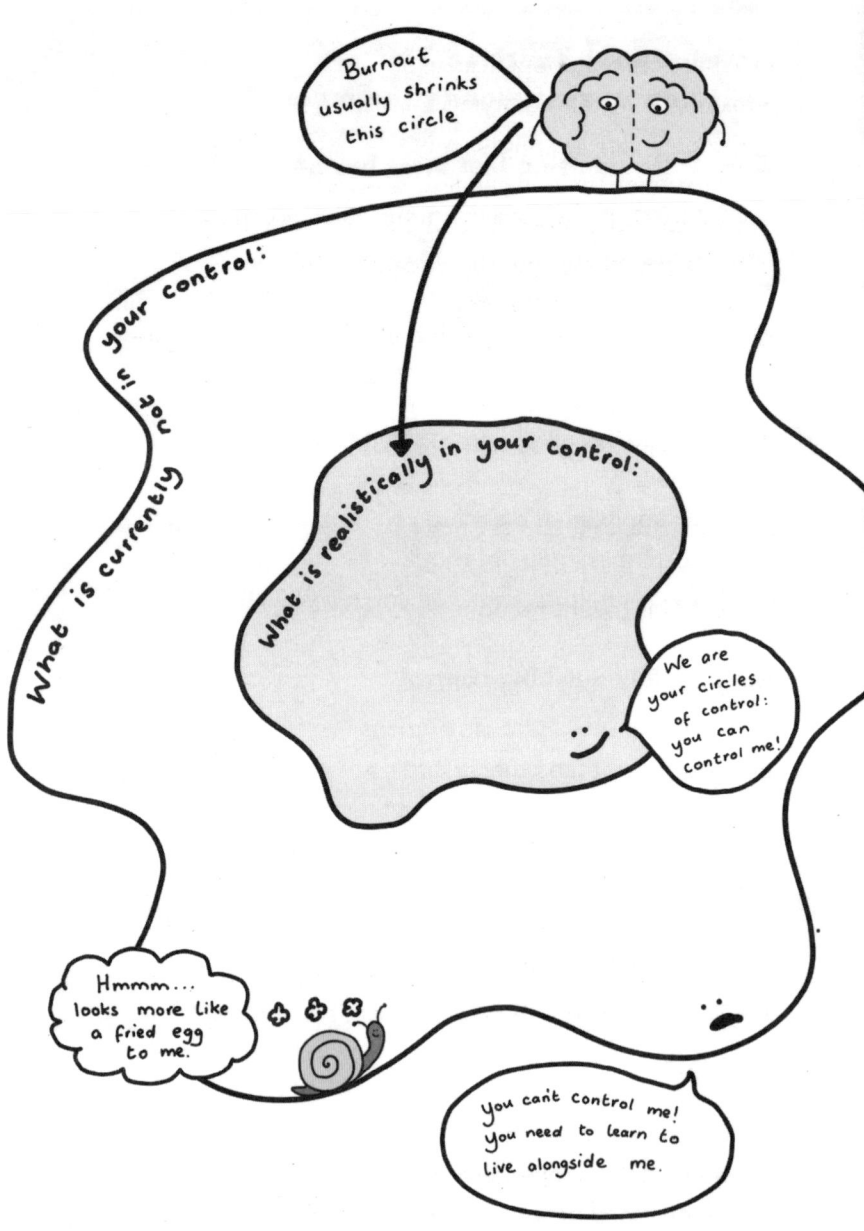

- Where can you beneficially focus your energy? For example, instead of trying to tidy the whole house (outer circle) you might want to do something smaller in the inner circle: clean a sock drawer, organize your calendar or work out a plan for something that's bothering you. This can give you a sense of achievement and control.

As you recover from burnout, it is likely your circle of control will grow. However, no one can control it all, and trying to is just another burnout trap!

Step 3: Learning to rest among the mess

It's critical to learn to rest among the mess burnout has created. This means recognizing that you don't have to be fully in control to enjoy yourself and you don't have to expend all your energy on getting back in control (what does that even mean?) before you can switch off. The problem isn't that the mess is stopping you from resting, the problem is that you BELIEVE you can't rest until you have controlled the perceived mess. During burnout, being able to rest and feel good is more important than being in control. These things can and will be tackled – when you have time and energy. But to have the energy you need to rest. NOW. Among the mess.

Think about:

- How can you help yourself switch off and rest even when there's still perceived mess?
- Are there any beliefs you need to challenge to allow yourself to do this?

- What can you do or say to give yourself permission to rest among the mess?
- If this is a physical mess, and seeing it makes you feel stressed, is there anything you need to do to help you switch off? Could you:
    - Create cosy corners where you can switch off?
    - Bung things in a cupboard?
    - Tackle one small thing then rest?
    - Remind yourself that sorting this will take time, but you need to enjoy yourself regardless?

Life Pathway 7: Replacing habits that harm

Your brain is in lower-power mode. New learning is effortful, and your brain will slip into habitual ways to maintain energy. This might be old habits that re-emerge or current habits that become more prominent. In normal, non-burned-out times, these habits may comfort and soothe – a quick break on your phone, a snack, purchasing a few goodies online. There is nothing inherently wrong with these. However, burned-out brains fall into habits more easily and have more difficulty getting out of them. These habits can keep us stuck, stop us finding paths out and even push us further into burnout.

My digital habit of mindlessly scrolling on my phone occurred more frequently when I was in low power mode, and it was harder to break the habit. Worst of all, it stopped me doing beneficial things, such as getting to sleep, and made me feel worse. You might blame yourself or your lack of willpower for getting stuck in habits, but this is actually about a lack of energy and cognitive resources. I see this as our brains' way of saving energy: it's trying to help you, but it's getting you stuck further.

Piecing your life back together after burnout

Just like we can't blame willpower for getting us there, we equally can't rely on willpower to get us out. This would require energy and resources we just don't have when burned out. Instead, we have to create barriers that stop us falling into these habits.

Let me explain: checking my phone at night kept me in high-alert mode. Trying to rely on willpower by keeping my phone by my bedside meant I needed to inhibit my habitual response to pick it up. Overriding or inhibiting behaviour requires lots of energy and cognitive resources. When in low-power mode, our brains will go for the least energy-consuming task – the habit. Therefore, relying on willpower meant I was likely to fail, as my brain wanted to habitually pick up the phone. Instead, I needed to create a barrier to make it harder for my brain to perform the habit. In this case, the barrier was leaving my phone downstairs and instead having a book beside my bed (an alternative habit to fill the gap). Now the response that required more energy was going to get my phone, and the book was an easier and more habitual response. Only by creating a barrier could I reduce this habit. I did the same for certain apps that were pulling me in and leaving me stressed – Instagram, for one. The barrier was taking it off my phone, so I had to switch on my computer if I wanted to check it, which required exerting more energy. It's even better if you can have a more helpful alternative to fill this habit gap, such as having a cuppa instead of checking Instagram.

Anti-burnout Exercise 32:
Building boulders to help shift habit paths

Think about which habits you fall into that make you feel worse. Instead of relying on willpower, think up some barriers you can create to stop you falling into habitual responses. If you can have an alternative that's easy to fill the gap, then this can push you along a more helpful habitual path to help you out of burnout.

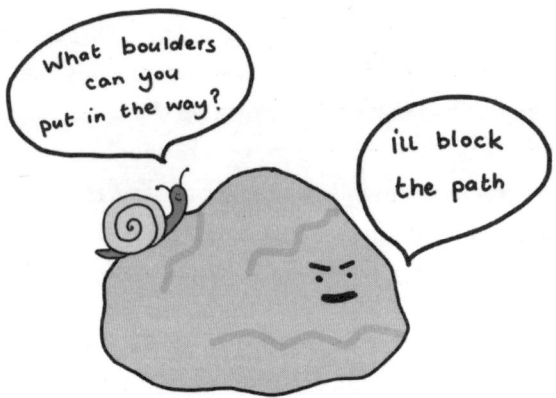

1. Habit I want to change
2. Barrier boulder I can put in the way of this habit
3. Alternative habit to fill this gap.

Anti-burnout takeaways

- Burnout can shrink your life so you no longer take part in activities or see people that are meaningful to you.
- Burnout can rupture your life path and you may feel grief for what you have lost or for your anticipated future.
- Burnout can also make you feel like you have lost your identity.
- Burnout can lead to mess – both metaphorical and physical. Life can feel messy, we can feel like a mess and there may be real mess surrounding us.
- The impact of burnout can make us feel like we have lost control.

7 Life Pathways out of burnout

- Pathway 1: Don't quash what you want and need.
- Pathway 2: Put some jigsaw pieces of yourself back together.
- Pathway 3: Regrow your roots and reconnect with the world.
- Pathway 4: Recapture joy, awe, wonder.
- Pathway 5: Rest is power.
- Pathway 6: Embrace the messiness.
- Pathway 7: Replace habits that harm.

Chapter 12
Building back stronger

You have taken the first few steps out of burnout – you can see there is a way forward. You are defrosting from your time in the arctic outpost, becoming a bit more alive, a little bit stronger, and hope glows brighter as you see that a future is possible. The paths ahead have become easier to find, but recovery is never a linear line: often progress is slow, we still take missteps and go backwards as well as forwards. The slow, gradual shifts can make us question if we really are making progress. If you look over your shoulder, you are can still see the outpost and it makes you afraid: if you slip back too far, will you return to full zombie mode? Your flame is gradually returning but you question if you are just retracing your steps to return to a place that will extinguish it again. The memory of burnout is still singed in patterns upon your neurons, indelibly it seems, and is activated easily, igniting fear that we are returning to that place. Knowing that burnout has wreaked havoc on your brain, body and life makes you fearful. Can you really build back? Is part of you perpetually lost or damaged? Will you ever feel like yourself again? Will burnout ever truly be part of your history rather than an omnipresent memory? Newsflash: you can recover, as evidenced by millions of ex-zombies that have gone before you.

Building back stronger

Good news from the ex-zombie army

As I write this, I look out the window to torrential rain battering the plants in my garden, knowing that that this will only make them grow back stronger and thrive. The research tells us that people can also move through dark times, recover, develop and even find ways to live that work better.[1] We have already read that in the BBC podcast *Illuminated: In Pieces*, burnout is described as 'an invitation to stop and think and create what you want out of the pieces,'[2] and recovery is when you do this. Many people describe experiencing post-traumatic growth[3] after difficult times, including greater appreciation of what we have, greater empathy, clarity about what matters and certainty in what we want, along with less judgement and the knowledge we can face challenges and come through them.

In my work, I have heard this many times. People say some version of 'I wish I had never experienced this, but I have come out better and I wouldn't change that.' I, too, wish I hadn't burned out, but if I hadn't, I would never have made certain changes in my life, or re-evaluated where I used my time, or shifted my metric of success. Like the plants in my garden, we can grow, thrive and live again. What's more, by finding ways out of the dark times we can strengthen the very core of our tree, develop stronger roots and train our branches to manage the weight in a different way. By coming through a storm, we can stop, evaluate life and decide where we want to grow next. Not only we can survive tough times, we can also build back better.

The art of recovery

Recovery isn't incidental: building back is an intentional act that requires our attention and resources. In his book *Recovery*,[4] Dr Gavin Francis says:

I often remind my patients that it's worth giving adequate time, energy and respect to the process of healing.

We can't rush recovery: if we push on without considering, pausing and noticing, we fail to notice we are on a circular route returning us to the start. Recovery is a skill, an art that we need to learn. It's not something to get right or to conquer – so abandon these pressures. Instead, it's something we need to get curious about, that we need to explore and learn from. There isn't a formulaic or marketed solution, it's a personal approach that requires getting to know ourselves better, including the parts we want to avoid, and working out what works for us.

Some of you will have recovered before, perhaps from illness or grief, and you can take this learning and use it here. For many of us it's unfamiliar terrain that we are exploring and discovering. We are beginners, learning something new and that brings discomfort, mistakes and setbacks. But this can't make us turn away – discomfort is an inevitable part of the process, and mistakes and setbacks give us valuable information about where to go next. Retreating from these just gets us stuck. Author Hannah Walker-Brown sums this up perfectly:

Recovery is messy, non-linear, but deeply creative.[5]

Recovery is not just an internal process; the external environment heals us too. We can use this knowledge to aid recovery by seeking circumstances, connections and spaces that enhance growth rather than hinder it.

Finding your new path

Being anti-burnout is recognizing that recovery is not just a return on the pathway to the place we were at before; it's identifying that another way is possible. It's not just learning, it's unlearning. It's not just building back our lives, it's dismantling the parts that never served us. It's not just getting stronger, it's learning to live with our vulnerabilities. It's taking a route that we choose rather than ambling mindlessly along the paths life pushes and pulls us. It's about designing a life that works for you.

One of the top five regrets of the dying, shared by author Bronnie Ware[6] from her experience as a palliative nurse, is:

I wish I'd had the courage to live a life true to myself, not a life others expected.

Burnout gives us the opportunity to do just that. As life shrinks and breaks down, we have the chance to reflect and rebuild life into something more meaningful and manageable. Yes, the experience may have fundamentally changed us, but that can be something to celebrate. I took these powerful words by Hannah Walker-Brown with me everywhere, typed in my phone, to remind me of this during my recovery from burnout. She tells us that recovery is:

Rejecting the idea that when we fall apart ... we are broken, when actually sometimes the wreckage brings us home.

The pathways in this chapter require a bit more energy and resources than the previous steps: they are for when you have regained some energy and are starting to move out of burnout. You now need to find ways to build back to a place that works for you, while ensuring that you don't just return to the same place that pushed you into burnout in the first instance. These paths are about helping your tree grow stronger roots, more supportive structural branches and creating more favourable external circumstances, so your tree can regenerate, grow back more resistant and even start to bloom.

7 Rebuilding Pathways out of burnout

Rebuilding Pathway 1: Knowledge and awareness

Being in the arctic outpost and inhabiting a zombie brain may have felt like a wasteland, but actually it was time to reflect and learn: it was instilling knowledge and giving you critically important information. For many of us, not having this information before was part of what led us to fall so deep into burnout – we didn't know we were getting there, and we didn't even notice we were there. We now know the signs we are starting to degenerate into zombies, and it's critical we use this information. This knowledge is power.

When we notice the telltale signs, instead of fearing we are stepping backwards into burnout, we can notice the dip and take action to climb out of it, rather than it becoming a chasm of burnout. If we do ever reach the outpost again, instead of wallowing there unaware, we can notice when we are there and take quick steps out. As we have already trodden the paths out, we know exactly where to look for them. By falling into burnout, we have been gifted with knowledge and awareness, so let's make sure we use it.

Building back stronger

Anti-burnout Exercise 33: Noticing the dips

Understanding our own signs helps us be aware we are entering a dip and use this knowledge to navigate ourselves out. The signs can be shifts in our thinking and cognition, emotions and behaviours. My signs are that my creativity starts to wane; I stop having ideas and lose enthusiasm. I also feel overwhelmed more often; the old beliefs start to whisper; I fall into unhelpful habits (the phone may even creep back into the bedroom!); I start to withdraw from root-fertilizing activities.

What your dips look like will be personal to you. The more you understand them, the more you can spot them and take action. Use the image below to think about the signs you are in a dip and which actions will get you out.

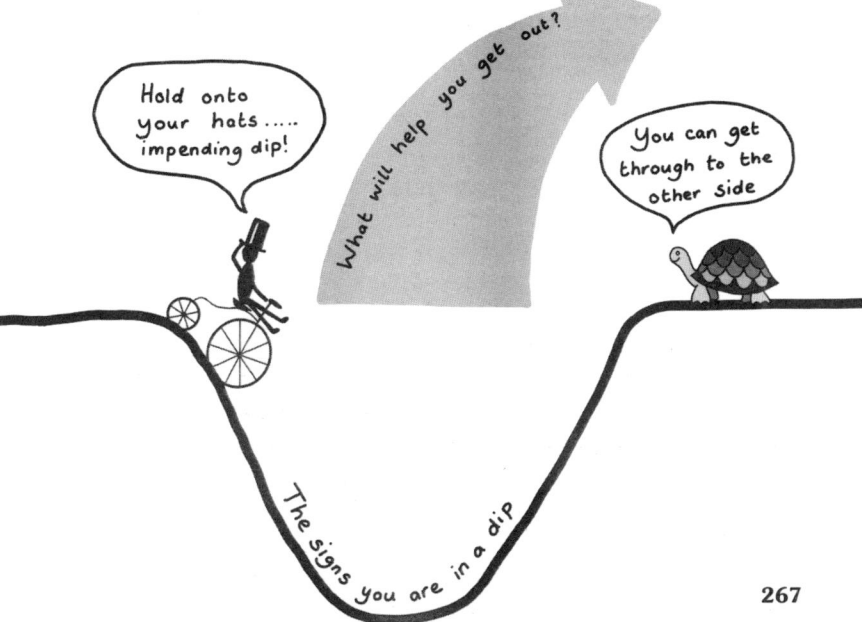

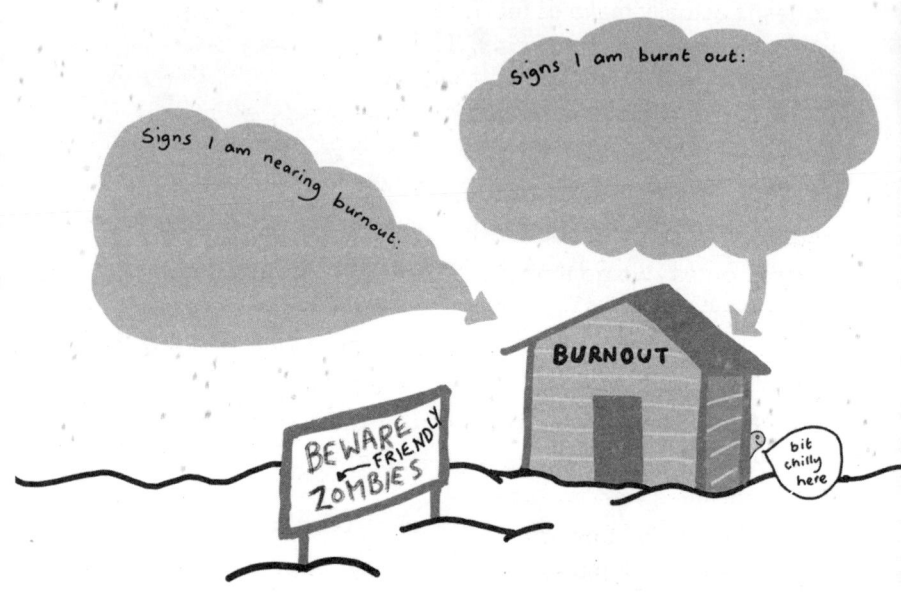

It's also important to understand the indicators that you are reaching or have reached the arctic outpost, so you can take quick, early action if you find yourself there again. Use the image to understand your indicators.

Rebuilding Pathway 2: Redefining your metrics of success

From an early age, we are indoctrinated into defining success with external indicators: our achievements, status, grades, promotions, wealth, possessions and productivity. We spend much of our energy trying to achieve these metrics of success, thinking that getting there (yes, it's another mythical THERE!) will help us feel happy or complete. The ironic findings of the research are that these beliefs are more likely to drive us into burnout and that striving for or even reaching these goals doesn't actually make us feel good – that lies elsewhere (more of that later).[7]

We need to unpick the metrics of success that we have been working towards in order to create our own (more helpful) definition of success. In her book *The Success Myth*[8] Emma Gannon talks about two phases (I'm going to call these 'routes') we go through in life (based on coach Donna Lancaster's work[9]):

- **Route 1** is a fast-paced motorway, following what we think we want and pursuing societies' traditional definition of success, for example, wealth and status. I envisage this route filled with obstacles and frequent slip roads: many people hit an obstacle or come off at some point. We need to go through Route 1 to get to Route 2 (although not everyone will get there).
- **Route 2** is about unlearning Route 1 and deciding what you really want, what your own metrics of success are. I like to think of burnout as a slip road that has rapidly taken us off Route 1 to the arctic outpost. It seems like we have derailed, but actually it has brought us to a fork in the road where we have a choice. We can go back up the slip road onto Route 1, or we can rethink how we operate and find Route 2 instead. Route 2 has a slower and more sustainable pace, aligned with your true values and your own metrics of success.

The Anti-Burnout Book

Anti-burnout Exercise 34: Redefining your metric of success

Use the image to think about what your Route 1 metrics of success were. Now think about how you want to define success for Route 2.

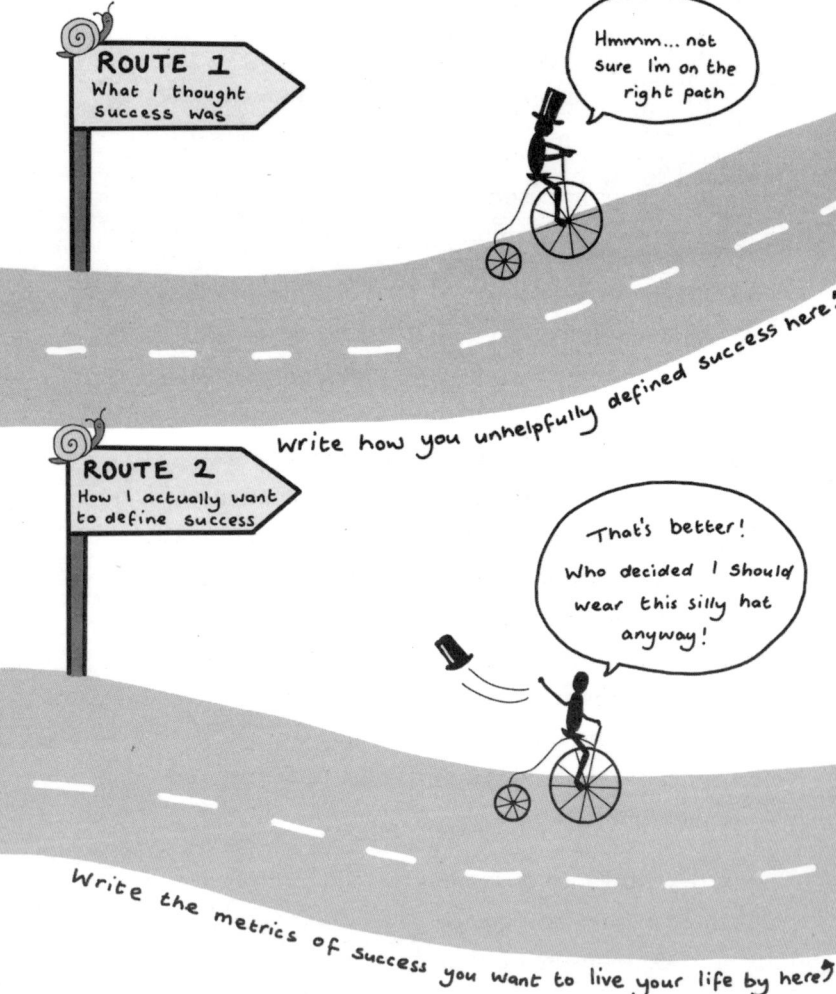

Rebuilding Pathway 3: Hanging your values in balance on your tree

You are now about to do something unexpected – add more weight to your tree. But this weight is beneficial, as it helps your tree know in which direction to grow, if we use your values wisely.

Values are what is meaningful to you, the qualities you want to grow your life around. We know that setting goals, taking action and living life when aligned with your values can make you feel good and improve wellbeing.[10] It's not just YOUR values that are important, it's the values in the environment around your tree. If these clash with your own values, it creates stress and can make you feel devalued, putting you more at risk of burnout.[11] Values are used frequently in clinical work, to help people with decisions, setting goals and building a life that works for them, particularly after difficult times. We probably all have a rough idea of our values but really understanding them and hanging them on your tree so they are displayed clearly can be helpful. We'll do this in the exercise below.

However, there's a caveat, and it relates to why I burned out. Sometimes just knowing our values isn't enough. I have always been values-driven, but it was a clash of my values, and adhering too strongly to certain values to the detriment of others, that led to me becoming burned out. My value was helping others, but by doing this too much, I overlooked the value of caring for myself. We need to balance our values and ensure we are tending to them all, and at times (for example when our capacity shrinks) we may need to prioritize certain values over others.

To ensure we balance our values, we can categorize how we place them in our tree. Those high up are the values we need to adhere to, to ensure our tree continues to grow upwards.

The low-lying fruit are also important to us, but to ensure they don't pull our tree down they need to be balanced with the high fruit. Ultimately, if we ignore the high fruit and only focus on the low fruit, this adds weight and pulls us down. So, when we think about values, we need to categorize them to ensure the balance is right. Let's start hanging fruit on your tree.

> ### Anti-burnout Exercise 35:
> ### Hanging your values on your tree
>
> **Step 1: Choosing your value apples.** Time to really think about your values. I have provided some apples in the basket that you can pick to add to your tree. This is not a comprehensive list but you can it as a starting point. List everything that is important to you from these values. Now select just a handful of the most important ones to add to your tree.
>
> **Step 2: Categorizing and hanging your values apples.** There are two categories: high fruit and low fruit. Select the values that are most important to you. If you had to prioritize just a handful of values, which would they be? These are your high fruit. You need to give time and focus to living your life around the high fruit to enable you to also tend to the low-lying fruit. Now think about which values can start to create stress if you put too much emphasis on them, without tending to your high-value fruit. These are your low-lying fruit – they are important too, but if you focus only on these, they will pull your tree downwards. You need to ensure there is balance to keep your tree healthy. Now add your values to the tree in two categories: high fruit and low fruit.

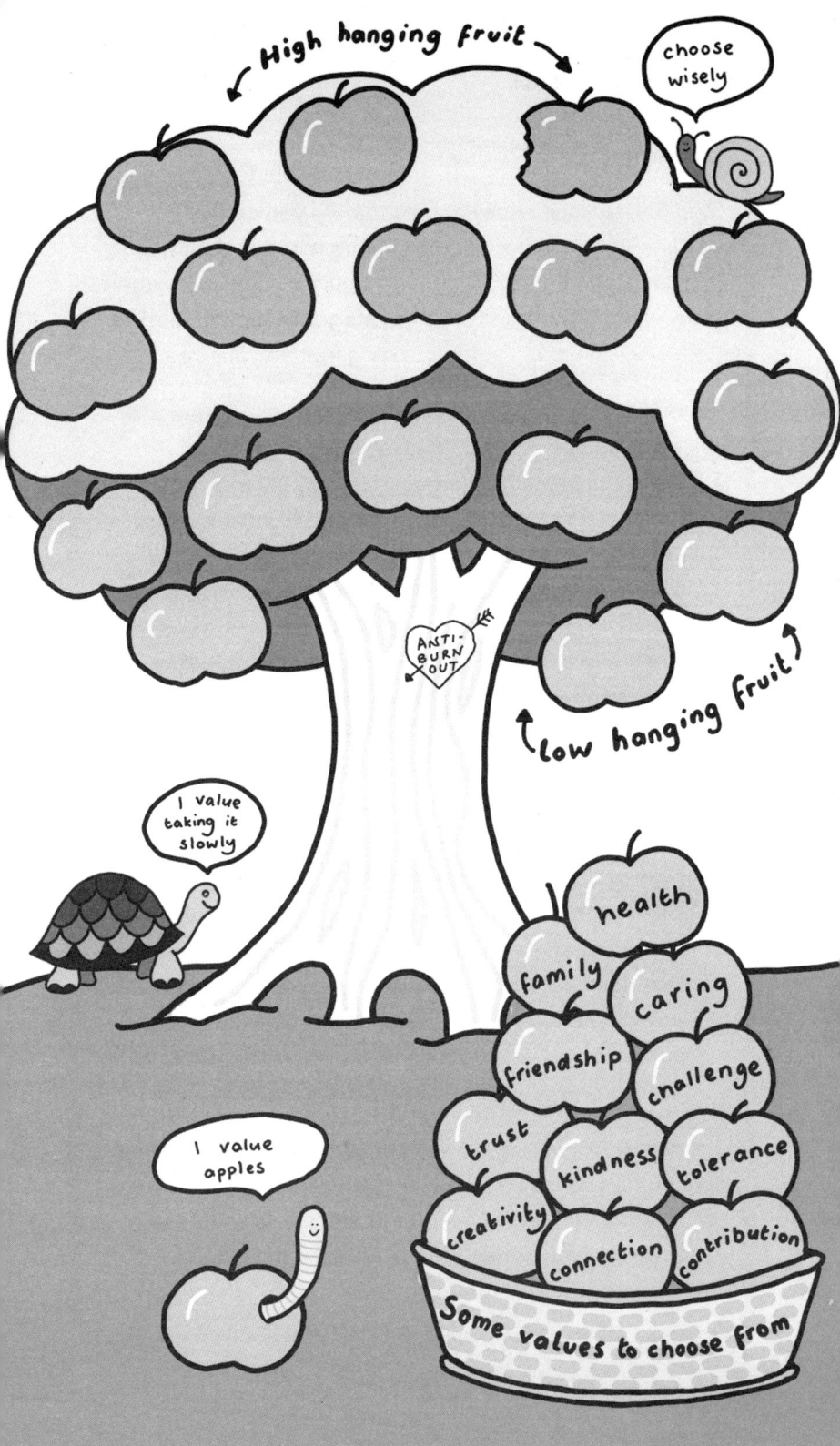

Step 3: Use your values apples to help you grow. Now you know your values and have hung them on your tree in balance, it's important you use these to help your tree grow in the right direction. Here are some ways to do this:

1. Think about how you can align your journey out of burnout with your values. Are your goals aligned with your values?
2. Are there values you are neglecting? What do you need to do to ensure you are including these values in your life? Is there anything you have to stop or give up (this could be beliefs, such as perfectionism) to ensure you can work towards these values?
3. Are you putting too much weight on certain values to the detriment of others? Are you enacting these values in one area of your life and not another (for example, in work but not at home)? What do you need to do to rebalance this?
4. Use your tree to make decisions. Which decisions align most with your high-value fruit?
5. Use your tree to think about what in your environment is causing stress and why. Are there things happening that don't align with your values? Does the environment stop you being able to act within your values? Does your context make you feel valued? What actions do you need to take around this?

Values are something we have to revisit regularly they can shift and it's easy to be knocked off paths. They can also sound simple, but I have found in my clinical work that really determining these and using them effectively in life can be complex. You may want to spend some more time

> really thinking about your values – I have included Further Reading on page 306 if you want to explore further. Also, don't forget to ensure you value yourself in the middle of it all!

Rebuilding Pathway 4: Commit to your non-negotiables

Much of life requires flexibility – your tree needs to bend in the wind – but on this pathway you are going to stand firm. Your non-negotiables are the foundations you need to continue functioning well. They are things that need to be set in stone, as much as you possibly can, throughout your days, weeks and life. Being clear on what these are helps you build your life around them, plan for them, remove barriers to doing them and set boundaries around them. Looking after your foundations helps keep you healthy and gives you more capacity to manage life.

I was terrible at having non-negotiables before burnout, but now I am steadfast in ensuring I stick to these as much as I can. Yes, sometimes they slip – and it's important not to let your inner critic take over when this happens. What's important is maintaining a long-term pattern of adhering to them: a few occasional deviations shouldn't push you off-track; however, bigger shifts can indicate you are off-course. Here are some of my non-negotiables, before you think of yours. Looking at my list, you may think, 'Really, that's so basic?' but it gives you an idea of what I was letting slip before I burned out. If you think about what contributed to your burnout, I suspect basic things will have been neglected too!

- **Eat breakfast:** I was shocking at eating this before burnout. I now find ways to ensure this happens, which might mean an easy breakfast option or prepping the night before.
- **Stop for lunch:** Yes, really! And preferably not at my desk. As much as possible, I block this time off on my calendar.
- **Leave a gap of at least 15 minutes between meetings:** I used to say 'yes' to any meeting time and rush from meeting to meeting. I don't always have control over this, but when I do, I stick to this rule.
- **Move daily:** It doesn't have to be big but it has to happen.
- **Take pockets of rest:** Planned throughout the day. While writing this book, it meant ensuring I had regular restful breaks and didn't just push through.
- **Prioritize sleep:** This means setting a good routine, leaving my phone out of the bedroom and putting in place activities that help me get to sleep at nighttime.
- **Make time for medical regimes:** This includes taking any necessary medication and monitoring and addressing symptoms, and it has to happen to stay healthy.

Now over to you. Keep these handy so you can check in with yourself regularly.

Brian the Brain reflections

- What are your non-negotiables?
- How can you ensure you adhere to these as much as possible?
- Do you need to do anything to prepare yourself to be able to implement these? This can be things like learning good sleep practices, creating restful spaces, buying equipment for making easy breakfasts

> (I'm thinking of my smoothie maker!) or learning digital skills to block off time or set meeting times in advance.
> - How can you notice when you fall off-track?

Rebuilding Pathway 5: The self-preservation society

The 'Self-preservation Society' is a song from the 1960s' film *The Italian Job*. I haven't seen it, but for some reason it's one of my many random earworms, which include 1970s' TV themes and 1980s' adverts. The song certainly wasn't designed to start a revolution against burnout, but that's how I use it now. It's not really a society with just one member, so I want to invite you to be a member of the self-preservation society.

I'm afraid there is an initiation before you are admitted to the society. It might seem a bit onerous to go through the process, but I promise you that once you have done this small bit of work to become a fully-fledged member, then it becomes a lot easier, and you will be less likely to fall into burnout. If you've decided on your non-negotiables, then you have already completed the first step (if not, go back and do it). Well done - now there are two more to go before you can join the society:

Initiation Step 1: No, no, no, no, no, no (to always saying yes)

Do you say 'yes' when you mean 'no'? Do you worry about saying no and think it will have a catastrophic effect? Does guilt make you say yes? Do you say yes too readily then feel overwhelmed, stressed and resentful by the things you have taken on? If you said yes too readily to these questions, then you must get through this initiation step to join the society:

learn to pause before saying yes and allowing yourself to say no.

You might need to do some groundwork to shift those old beliefs (my letting people down, for example) to enable you to do this. To join the society, you need to agree to follow this doctrine:

> **I agree to the yes/no decision doctrine:**
>
> When you feel the urge to say yes, STOP and pause before you do.
>
> If you need to think further, you can always use a holding message at this point if needed. This might include:
>
> - I'll need to check my schedule.
> - I am not sure I have capacity to take this on right now, but I will get back to you.
> - Let me have a think before I get back to you.
>
> Now you are at a decision point, with three choices: yes, no or unsure. To make these decisions, think about the following:
>
> - How do you feel about the decision?
> - What are the consequences of saying yes or no?
> - Will this be detrimental in any way? If so, are you willing to accept the consequences?
> - What would saying no allow you to do instead?
> - What will saying yes stop you doing?
> - What would you advise someone else to do?
>
> Hopefully you have now come to a decision of yes or no.

However, if you are still unsure, follow the unsure pathway so you can interrogate this a bit more.

Yes: This should only be a choice if you have capacity, if you want to say yes and if it will not be detrimental to your wellbeing; or, if you recognize it may be detrimental but you are able to live with any consequences.

No: If you find this hard, then have stock phrases prepared. You can even do this proactively by setting an automatic reply message in your email when you notice you are at full capacity. Here are some stock replies I use:

- Thanks so much for thinking of me, I'm sorry I don't have the space to take this on right now.
- I would really love to join you (I only say this if it's true!), however I can't make it on this occasion. Hopefully I can make future events/we can arrange something soon.
- I'm really sorry, I don't have the time right now to do this justice, however, have you considered ... x,y,z [possible alternatives].

Unsure: Interrogate the decision. It can be helpful to write this down or talk it through with someone you trust. These questions can also be helpful:

- What decision fits with balancing your values tree?
- What decision fits with your new metric of success?
- How do these decisions impact your capacity, energy and stress levels?
- What are you worried will happen if you say no? Is this realistic?

Well done! You've passed this part of the initiation ceremony. To remain in the society, you need to continue to pause and consider whether the no option is better, when you feel the urge to say yes.

Initiation Step 2: Protecting your precious resources

Now for the next stage of initiation – get through this and you are part of the gang. You may call them boundaries, I call them protecting your precious resources, because that's what we are doing. We are valuing and protecting our resources of time, energy, capacity, emotions, values and material goods. By valuing and protecting our resources, we shift from being depleted by things which don't really matter to conserving our energy and using it wisely on the activities and people who matter – yourself included! We've already started one of the first steps towards this: learning to say no so we can make informed yeses.

Protecting your resources can feel weird at first: you may be used to thinking of the needs of others before your own. You may be scared of the potential consequences. Protecting your resources sometimes requires significant behaviour shifts, such as asserting your needs, expressing what you think and feel, and of course saying no. This can trigger old beliefs ('I am selfish,' 'I am letting people down'). There will be discomfort and most likely difficult feelings (hello shame and guilt!). There may well be consequences: people may lose interest when you are no longer perpetually serving their needs, and opportunities may have to be passed up. However, it is usually the things that don't matter so much that fall to the wayside, leaving space for what does matter. For all the awkwardness and potential collateral damage, the outcome normally has far more benefits than downsides.

Protecting your resources is anything but selfish; it enables you to care better for others and really prioritize those things and people that matter. You have more capacity and energy to tackle what's important and create change. It's not about switching off from world and social issues, it's about setting boundaries so the action you take is more powerful. It can take work, but the work is worth it.

> **Anti-burnout Exercise 36:**
> **A commitment to preserve your precious resources**
>
> Using the prompts below, think about how to protect your precious resources. These could include the following areas: **time**, **energy**, **values**, **emotions** and **physical resources** (e.g. space, money).
>
> For each area of your resources think about the following:
>
> - What drains your resources most?
> - Does anything drain your resources unnecessarily?
> - Do you find yourself often agreeing to things that drain you? What are they?
> - What do you feel pressure to do?
> - What do you need to do to protect your resources?
>
> What are three simple things you can do going forward to commit to protecting your resources? Make a plan and a promise to yourself to keep up these three simple changes.

Joining the self-preservation society

Congratulations! You have passed your initiation and are a fully-fledged member of the self-preservation society. Really, though, this is about community and society preservation too – we are gifting ourselves the resources to focus on and tackle what matters, including the bigger issues. Now for your initiation bonus gift …

Bonus initiation gift: The 'F it!' bucket

Use this bucket as a quick reminder to yourself of what really matters. Didn't manage to do everything you meant to do today? Throw that thought in the bucket. Think you should bake a birthday cake from scratch? Throw it in the bucket and buy one from the shop. Concerned about how other people perceive you? Throw it in the bucket and work on sticking to your own values. A lot of the things that we tell ourselves are important just aren't. Your initiation gift is a reminder to stop wasting your energy on things that really don't matter and throw it in the bucket instead.

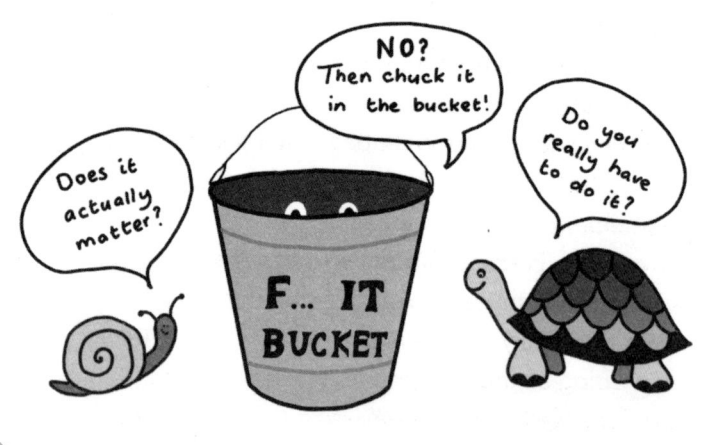

Rebuilding Pathway 6: Using reductions to grow (and what we always need to increase)

Reduce, slow down, reflect: All too often we think that to improve we need to have more, do more, achieve more or add more things in. However, the research tells us that the converse is true: we are more likely to make our life better by reducing, cutting back and slowing down. Feeling time-pressured and rushing just adds to the weight in our branches. Allowing ourselves time, reducing what we must do and removing time pressure makes us feel better.

Here are some suggestions for what you can reduce to help yourself grow:

- Remind yourself you have time. You are not wasting it. You do not have to rush. Just the simple statement 'I have time' can be enough to relax you.
- Reduce the pressure to use time well. What does this even mean? Challenge this belief and just let yourself be.
- Reduce what you do in a day. Don't set impossible 'to do' lists. Keep it simple.
- Reduce multi-tasking. Allow yourself to just focus on one thing.
- Reduce your material goods. This can be difficult for some people, and there's no moral value here, it's simply about having less information to sift through, visually and cognitively. Even one tiny area such as your kitchen drawer can help.
- Slow down. Practise mindfulness, meditation, yoga, meandering aimlessly or anything else that helps you slow down physically and mentally.
- Stop doing all the time and let yourself reflect. What have you done well? What hasn't worked for you? What are you proud of? How do you feel? What do you need?

- Stop striving for perfection and allow things to be good enough. Most things can use less energy and still have much the same effect if you let them be good enough – even yourself.

> **Brian the Brain reflections**
>
> - What reductions can you make?
> - How can you slow down?
> - How can you stop to reflect throughout your days/months/years?

There are, however, three fundamental factors that you shouldn't reduce. In fact, it's imperative you increase these as part of your route forward to strengthen your tree:

Social connection: Build, build, build your social connection to people who cheerlead and support you, who make you feel safe and energized, and who help you weather the storms. Good quality social connections are the strongest predictor of wellbeing – make time to build supportive relationships and networks at home and work. This isn't aways about socializing (too much can be draining) – it's about investing in connections.

Self-compassion: You can never have too much self-compassion. It reduces stress and helps you stay healthy and weather life's storms. Building compassion takes work and can be a life-long journey: I've included resources on page 306 to help you ensure this is part of your route. When talking about her self-compassion journey, author Elizabeth Gilbert said:

Think about what you need to hear, and speak to yourself like this again and again and again.

For now, start simple by being as generously kind to yourself as you are to others.

Accept support from others: We all need support and validation from those around us. Allowing ourselves to be helped is not some fundamental failure, it is an intrinsic factor that builds strong bonds and guides us through life. Accepting help from people around you enables you to utilize their billions of neurons, capacity, energy and perspectives to navigate the tough stuff, which is always easier when done collectively. It also strengthens bonds and is mutually beneficial for the helper and the helped. So, throw aside the burdensome belief of feeling like you are a burden and think about how you can accept help instead.

Have a think about how you might strengthen these three fundamental factors going forwards.

Rebuilding Pathway 7: When enough is enough – changing your environment

As our energy recovers, we often start to realize that we have been living with unacceptable weather around our tree. It wasn't a personal failure that we broke, it's that we had too much to carry and were trying to survive in conditions that didn't promote growth. This realization is freeing, but it comes with a challenge. That challenge is that something needs to change. We need to take action to change the circumstances (which might include toxic workplaces or toxic relationships), shift our tree into different surroundings or (in the worst-case scenario) find ways to cope until we can make more dramatic shifts.

Making change can be hard and feel risky, as we are moving from a known (albeit an unhelpful one) to an unknown. We can be unsure how to action this change as we have never done it before, or we can debate whether change is the best option, so we get stuck. There can be barriers, including financial ones, so we may need to build some groundwork before we induce change. Realizing that the environment needs to change is a positive step, but enacting the change we know we need isn't always easy. Below are some ideas to help.

**Anti-burnout Exercise 37:
What to do when your situation needs to change**

Clearly identify the issue

1. What is the specific issue in your context/environment?
2. What would you like to be different? Envisage what this would look like. What would it feel like?

Work out what can be changed

3. Can the context be changed to help your tree or do you need to move your tree into a different context?
4. What are the barriers in place to changing the context? Can it realistically be changed?
5. What support could help you work through change? Maybe talking therapy, finding a work mentor, opening up to someone you trust.
6. What are the risks to doing something different? What are the risks to staying put?

How to make this change

7. What are the possible solutions? Write them all down and explore which solution is best. Can you get support to think through this?
8. What is the best solution to try first? What is the first step to putting this in place? Can you plan the next steps after this? Try to be as concrete and specific as possible about the steps you can take. Sometimes the next step won't emerge until you've completed another step.
9. If this doesn't work, what is the next best solution to try?

What to do if the context can't immediately be changed

10. Think about what you need to do to ensure you can survive in this context.
11. Is there any groundwork you need to do before you can change the context (such as exploring training/other possible roles, if you are thinking about changing jobs)?

Change is always hard, and we often need support. But recognizing what you want to change and thinking about how you can do it focuses you on that route forwards.

The Anti-Burnout Book

Anti-burnout takeaways

- Recovery is possible from burnout and many people report growth and a positive change after it.
- Building back is not just about putting the pieces of your life back together, it is also about deciding what you want to leave behind.
- Building back is not returning on the same path; it's creating new paths that are more sustainable long term.
- Recovery is not a linear progression; we will take missteps and go backwards as well as going forwards. It requires time, patience and creativity.
- Once you have taken the first steps out of burnout, continuing along the paths requires a bit more energy to create sustainable long-term lifestyle changes.
- Building back is about designing a life that works for you which is less likely to return you to burnout.

7 Rebuilding Pathways out of burnout

- Pathway 1: Use your knowledge and awareness.
- Pathway 2: Redefine your metrics of success.
- Pathway 3: Hang your values in your tree.
- Pathway 4: Commit to your non-negotiables.
- Pathway 5: Join the self-preservation society.
- Pathway 6: Reduce to grow.
- Pathway 7: Know when enough is enough.
- Multiple bonus pathways: Now you are moving out of burnout, you can use any of the proactive anti-burnout strategies in Chapters 1–8 to continue creating anti-burnout pathways out and building an anti-burnout life going forward.

Conclusion

Congratulations! Now that you have completed this book you are a fully-fledged founding member of the anti-burnout gang. No, make that revolution. Whether you are a current zombie, ex-zombie or trying to avoid burnout for yourself or other people, you now have a responsibility to take this forward in your own life. Grab your badge and wear it with pride, and use the knowledge you have gained to influence positively your life and the lives of those around you.

Being in the anti-burnout gang isn't about becoming invincible, that's not realistic. It's about carrying what we have learned with us to face the inevitable challenges that life brings. Life isn't there for the conquering: it's an ebb and flow of good times and not-so-good times, feeling great and feeling not-so great. Being anti-burnout is about learning what works and unlearning what doesn't work, to both protect ourselves and make our lives work better for us. If we find ourselves in an ebb (or even at the arctic outpost), then we need to recognize where we are, see it is as just part of life and ensure we utilize our skills to find the pathways out.

In addition, there is no formulaic one-size-fits-all way to be in the anti-burnout gang. What works for you will be unique to your mix of personality, preferences and situation: most members will need to experiment to find the right mix for them. Being in the anti-burnout gang is about testing out what works, which requires a willingness to get things wrong, to learn what is right for you. Finally, being anti-burnout is not a quick fix, it's ongoing, sometimes difficult, work that can involve dismantling long-term beliefs and behaviours. It may feel tough at times, but the effort and energy expenditure is worth it, because it improves our lives long-term.

The best thing about being in the anti-burnout gang is that you are never alone. This is a great big gang of past, present and trying-not-to-be future zombies who can support each other to be anti-burnout. Find your fellow members and utilize this support because collectively we are a powerful anti-burnout force that can help each other get out and stay out of burnout.

Go forth and be anti-burnout in your life, but also spread the message far and wide so we can build an anti-burnout world for as many people as possible.

Notes

Introduction

1   Caspi, A, Houts, R M, Ambler, A et al (2020). Longitudinal assessment of mental health disorders and comorbidities across four decades among participants in the Dunedin birth cohort study. *JAMA Network Open*, 3(4).
2   Gannon, E (2026). *A Year of Nothing*. Whitefox Publishing Limited.
3   May, K (2020). *Wintering: The power of rest and retreat in difficult times*. Rider.
4   Of note here is that how burnout is measured may vary across different surveys, leading to different rates of burnout being reported across studies. The most accurate will use a validated measure such as the Maslach Burnout Inventory, which has been validated for use in lots of different groups and is based on a definition of burnout.
5   www.deloitte.com/southeast-asia/en/issues/work/content/genz-millennialsurvey.html
    www2.deloitte.com/us/en/pages/about-deloitte/articles/burnout-survey.html
6   Gawlick, K & Mazurek Melnyk, B (2022). Examining the Epidemic of Working Parental Burnout and Strategies to Help: Ohio State University.

Chapter 1: What is burnout? And how do I know it's happened?

1   World Health Organization (2022). ICD-11: International classification of diseases (11th revision). icd.who.int/ ICD-11 was announced in 2019 but came into effect in 2022.
2   Burnout was included in ICD-10 but in much less detail.
3   Schaufeli, W B (2017). Burnout: A Short Socio-Cultural History. In: Neckel, S, Schaffner, A, Wagner, G (eds) Burnout, Fatigue, Exhaustion. Palgrave Macmillan, Cham. doi.org/10.1007/978-3-319-52887-8_5
4   Freudenberger H J, Staff burnout. J Soc Issues (1974) 30:159–65. 10.1111/j.1540-4560.1974.tb00706.
5   www.nytimes.com/1999/12/05/nyregion/herbert-freudenberger-73-coiner-of-burnout-is-dead.html
6   Maslach, C (1976). Burned Out. *Human Behaviour, 5 (9), 16–22*.
    Schaufeli, W B, Leiter, M P, & Maslach, C (2009). Burnout: 35 years of research and practice. *Career Development International*, 14(3), 204–220.

291

7 Baumeister, R F, Bratslavsky, E, Finkenauer, C, & Vohs, K D (2001). Bad is stronger than good. *Review of General Psychology, 5*(4), 323–370. doi.org/10.1037/1089-2680.5.4.323
8 thehyphen.substack.com
9 katherinemay.substack.com
10 Schaufeli, W B, Desart, S, & De Witte, H (2020). Burnout Assessment Tool (BAT)-Development, Validity and Reliability. *International Journal of Environmental Research and Public Health, 17*(24), 9495. doi.org/10.3390/ijerph17249495
11 Ibid
12 Maslach C, Leiter M P, Jackson S E. Maslach Burnout Inventory Manual. 4th ed. Mind Garden, Inc.; Palo Alto, CA, USA: 2017.
13 Free-to-use assessment tools: burnoutassessmenttool.be/handleiding_vragenlijst_eng/
The Maslach Burnout inventory is available online for personal or professional use for a fee: www.mindgarden.com/332-maslach-burnout-toolkit-for-general-use
14 World Health Organization (2022). ICD-11: *International Classification of Diseases* (11th revision). icd.who.int/
15 hbr.org/2021/02/how-the-pandemic-exacerbated-burnout
16 Luke van der Laan, Gail Ormsby, Lee Fergusson, Peter McIlveen (2023). Is this work? Revisiting the definition of work in the 21st century. *Journal of Work-Applied Management* 27 15 (2): 252–272. doi.org/10.1108/JWAM-04-2023-0035
17 Seedat S, Rondon M. Women's wellbeing and the burden of unpaid work. BMJ. 2021 Aug 31;374:n1972. doi: 10.1136/bmj.n1972
18 Nancy Beauregard, Alain Marchand, Jaunathan Bilodeau, Pierre Durand, Andrée Demers, Victor Y Haines. Gendered Pathways to Burnout: Results from the SALVEO Study, (2018) *Annals of Work Exposures and Health*, Volume 62, Issue 4, May 2018, Pages 426–437, doi.org/10.1093/annweh/wxx114
19 assets.publishing.service.gov.uk/media/60ae4501d3bf7f7383db35fc/Unpaid-and-Unrecognised1.pdf
20 Bianchi, R, Manzano-García, G, & Rolland, J P (2021). Is Burnout Primarily Linked to Work-Situated Factors? A Relative Weight Analytic Study. *Frontiers in Psychology, 11*, 623912. doi.org/10.3389/fpsyg.2020.623912
21 Shirom, A, Melamed, S, Toker, S, Berliner, S and Shapira, I (2005). Burnout and Health Review: Current Knowledge and Future Research Directions. International Review of Industrial and Organizational Psychology 2005 (eds G P Hodgkinson and J K Ford). doi.org/10.1002/0470029307.ch7

22 Renzo Bianchi, Irvin Sam Schonfeld, Eric Laurent (2015). Burnout-depression overlap: A review, *Clinical Psychology Review*, 36, 28–41
23 Leclercq, C, & Hansez, I (2024). Temporal Stages of Burnout: How to Design Prevention? *International Journal of Environmental Research and Public Health*, 21(12), 1617. doi.org/10.3390/ijerph21121617
Hillert, A, Albrecht, A & Voderholzer, U (2020). The Burnout Phenomenon: A Résumé After More Than 15,000 Scientific Publications. *Frontiers in Psychiatry*, 11, 519237. doi.org/10.3389/fpsyt.2020.51923

Chapter 2: Building a burnout tree: Understanding what contributes to burnout

1 Bakker, et al (2023). Job demands-resources theory: Ten years later. *Annual Review of Organizational Psychology and Organizational Behaviour*, 10, 25–53. doi.org/10.1146/annurev-orgpsych-120920-053933
Bianchi, R, Manzano-García, G & Rolland, J P (2021). Is Burnout Primarily Linked to Work-Situated Factors? A Relative Weight Analytic Study. *Frontiers in Psychology*, 11, 623912. doi.org/10.3389/fpsyg.2020.623912
Shoman, et al (2021). Predictors of Occupational Burnout: A Systematic Review. *International Journal of Environmental Research and Public Health*, 18(17), 9188. doi.org/10.3390/ijerph18179188
Maslach, C and Leiter, M P (2016). Understanding the burnout experience: recent research and its implications for psychiatry. *World Psychiatry*, 15: 103–111. doi.org/10.1002/wps.20311
Mijakoski et al (2022). Determinants of Burnout Among Teachers: A Systematic Review of Longitudinal Studies. *International Journal of Environmental Research and Public Health*, 19(9), 5776. doi.org/10.3390/ijerph19095776
Chaves-Montero et al (2025). Analysis of the Predictors and Consequential Factors of Emotional Exhaustion Among Social Workers: A Systematic Review. *Healthcare*, 13(5), 552. doi.org/10.3390/healthcare13050552
Green, A E, Albanese, B J, Shapiro, N M, & Aarons, G A (2014). The roles of individual and organizational factors in burnout among community-based mental health service providers. *Psychological Services*, 11(1), 41–49. doi.org/10.1037/a0035299
Burnout_in_healthcare_risk_factors_and_solutions_July2023_0.pdf
2 Marchand, et al (2018). Do age and gender contribute to workers' burnout symptoms? *Occupational Medicine* (Oxford, England), 68(6), 405–411. doi.org/10.1093/occmed/kqy088

3   Artz, B, Kaya, I & Kaya, O (2022). Gender role perspectives and job burnout. *Review of Economics of the Household*, *20*(2), 447-470.
4   Turjeman-Levi, Y, Itzchakov, G & Engel-Yeger, B (2024). Executive function deficits mediate the relationship between employees' ADHD and job burnout. *AIMS public health*, *11*(1), 294-314.
    Arnold, S R, Higgins, J M, Weise, J, Desai, A, Pellicano, E & Trollor, J N (2023). Towards the measurement of autistic burnout. *Autism: The International Journal of Research and Practice*, *27*(7), 1933-1948.
    Schatz, D B & Rostain, A L (2006). ADHD with comorbid anxiety: a review of the current literature. *Journal of Attention Disorders*, *10*(2), 141-149.
5   Hill, A P & Curran, T (2016). Multidimensional Perfectionism and Burnout: A Meta-Analysis. Personality and Social Psychology Review, 20(3), 269-288.

Chapter 3: Under pressure: Stress, stress and more stress

1   Sandor Szabo, Yvette Tache & Arpad Somogyi (2012). The legacy of Hans Selye and the origins of stress research: A retrospective 75 years after his landmark brief 'Letter' to the Editor# of Nature, Stress, 15:5, 472-478, DOI: 10.3109/10253890.2012.710919
2   Zeynep et al (2024). Translational models of stress and resilience: An applied neuroscience methodology review, Neuroscience Applied, 3.
3   Campagne, D (2019). Stress and perceived social isolation (loneliness), Archives of Gerontology and Geriatrics, 82, 192-199.
4   Adam Bayes, Gabriela Tavella & Gordon Parker (2021). The biology of burnout: Causes and consequences, The World Journal of Biological Psychiatry, 22:9, 686-698.
5   Schneiderman, N, Ironson, G & Siegel, S D (2005). Stress and health: psychological, behavioural and biological determinants. *Annual Review of Clinical Psychology*, *1*, 607-628. doi.org/10.1146/annurev.clinpsy.1.102803.144141
6   Yaribeygi, H, Panahi, Y, Sahraei, H, Johnston, T P & Sahebkar, A (2017). The impact of stress on body function: A review. *EXCLI journal*, *16*, 1057-1072. doi.org/10.17179/excli2017-480
7   Lee, R S (2022). The physiology of stress and the human body's response to stress. In *Epigenetics of Stress and Stress Disorders* (pp1-18). Elsevier. doi.org/10.1016/B978-0-12-823039-8.00017-4
    Ghasemi, F, Beversdorf, D Q & Herman, K C (2024). Stress and stress responses: A narrative literature review from physiological mechanisms to intervention approaches. *Journal of Pacific Rim Psychology*, *18*. doi.org/10.1177/18344909241289222

Notes

8   See Lisa Feldman-Barret's books for more information: (2021). *Seven and a half lessons about the brain*. Mariner Books. Chicago/Turabian. (2017). *How emotions are made: The secret life of the brain*. Houghton Mifflin Harcourt.

9   Girotti, M, Bulin, S E & Carreno, F R (2024). Effects of chronic stress on cognitive function – From neurobiology to intervention. *Neurobiology of Stress*, *33*, 100670. doi.org/10.1016/j.ynstr.2024.100670
    Roberts, B L & Karatsoreos, I N (2021). Brain-body responses to chronic stress: a brief review. *Faculty Reviews*, *10*, 83. doi.org/10.12703/r/10-83

10 McEwen, B S (2017). Neurobiological and Systemic Effects of Chronic Stress. *Chronic stress (Thousand Oaks, Calif.)*, *1*, 2470547017692328. doi.org/10.1177/2470547017692328

11 Adam Bayes, Gabriela Tavella & Gordon Parker (2021). The biology of burnout: Causes and consequences, The World Journal of Biological Psychiatry, 22:9, 686-698, DOI: 10.1080/15622975.2021.1907713
    Arno van Dam (2021). A clinical perspective on burnout: diagnosis, classification and treatment of clinical burnout, European Journal of Work and Organizational Psychology, 30:5, 732-741, DOI: 10.1080/1359432X.2021.1948400
    Yaribeygi, H, Panahi, Y, Sahraei, H, Johnston, T P & Sahebkar, A (2017). The impact of stress on body function: A review. *EXCLI journal*, *16*, 1057-1072. doi.org/10.17179/excli2017-480
    Ghasemi, F, Beversdorf, D Q & Herman, K C (2024). Stress and stress resp0on, A L (2024). The utility of coping through emotional approach: A meta-analysis. *Health Psychology*, *43*(6), 397-417. doi.org/10.1037/hea0001364
    Shin, H, Park, Y M, Ying, J Y, Kim, B, Noh, H & Lee, S M (2014). Relationships between coping strategies and burnout symptoms: A meta-analytic approach. *Professional Psychology: Research and Practice*, *45*(1), 44-56. doi.org/10.1037/a0035220

Chapter 4: Beliefs and burnout

1   Connors, M H & Halligan, P W (2015). A cognitive account of belief: a tentative road map. *Frontiers in Psychology*, *5*, 1588. doi.org/10.3389/fpsyg.2014.0158

2   Agarwal, P (2022). *Hysterical: Exploding the Myth of Gendered Emotions*. Canongate Books.

3   Agarwal, P (2020). Sway: Unravelling Unconscious Bias. Bloomsbury Sigma.

4   Anna Katharina Schaffner (2024). *Exhausted: An A–Z for the Weary*. Profile Books.

5   Hill, A P & Curran, T (2016). Multidimensional Perfectionism and Burnout: A Meta-Analysis. *Personality and Social Psychology Review,* 20(3), 269–288.

Chapter 5: Let's get physical, and emotional

1   Hepburn, E (2023). *A toolkit for your emotions: 45 ways to feel better.* London: Greenfinch.
2   Glise, K, Wiegner, L & Jonsdottir, I H. Long-term follow-up of residual symptoms in patients treated for stress-related exhaustion. *BMC Psychol* 8, 26 (2020).
3   Trudel-Fitzgerald, C, Qureshi, F, Appleton, A A & Kubzansky, L D (2017). A healthy mix of emotions: underlying biological pathways linking emotions to physical health. *Current Opinion in Behavioural Sciences, 15,* 16–21. doi.org/10.1016/j.cobeha.2017.05.003
4   Ford, B Q, Lam, P, John, O P & Mauss, I B (2018). The psychological health benefits of accepting negative emotions and thoughts: Laboratory, diary and longitudinal evidence. *Journal of Personality and Social Psychology, 115*(6), 1075–1092. doi.org/10.1037/pspp0000157
5   De France, K & Hollenstein, T (2019). Emotion regulation and relations to wellbeing across the lifespan. *Developmental Psychology, 55*(8), 1768–1774. doi.org/10.1037/dev0000744
6   Rutherford, H J, Wallace, N S, Laurent, H K & Mayes, L C (2015). Emotion Regulation in Parenthood. *Developmental Review: DR, 36,* 1–14. doi.org/10.1016/j.dr.2014.12.008
7   Flores-Kanter, P E, Moretti, L & Medrano, L A (2021). A narrative review of emotion regulation process in stress and recovery phases. *Heliyon, 7*(6), e07218. doi.org/10.1016/j.heliyon.2021.e0
8   Sun, J, Wayne, S J & Liu, Y (2021). The Roller Coaster of Leader Affect: An Investigation of Observed Leader Affect Variability and Engagement. *Journal of Management, 48*(5), 1188–1213.
9   Cintron, D W & Ong, A D (2024). Trajectories of affective wellbeing and survival in middle-aged and older adults. *Emotion, 24*(5), 1149–1156. doi.org/10.1037/emo0001341
    Sadler, Miller, Christensen and McGue (2011). Subjective wellbeing and longevity: a co-twin control study. Twin Research and Human Genetics, 14 (3), 249–256.
10 Barrett, L F (2017). *How emotions are made: The secret life of the brain.* Houghton Mifflin Harcourt.

Notes

Chapter 6: Making work work for you: Let's take a look at your day job

1   Waddell & Burton (2006). Is Work Good for Your Health and Wellbeing? Executive Summary. London: The Stationary Office.
2   Stevenson, D & Farmer, P (2017). Thriving at Work: A Review of Mental Health and Employers [Report]. Department for Work and Pensions and Department of Health and Social Care.
3   2023 survey by The Workforce Institute at UKG. For a summary see: www.forbes.com/sites/tracybrower/2023/01/29/managers-have-major-impact-on-mental-health-how-to-lead-for-wellbeing
4   www.cipd.org/uk/knowledge/reports/health-well-being-work
5   For a summary of the data see: whatworkswellbeing.org/wp-content/uploads/2020/02/factsheet-why-invest-employee-wellbeing-may2017.pdf
6   Deloitte (2020). Mental health and employers: Refreshing the case for investment www2.deloitte.com/uk/en/pages/consulting/articles/mental-health-and-employers-refreshing-the-case-for-investment.html
7   Bragge, P, Delafosse, V, Kellner, P, Cong-Lem, N, Tsering, D, Giummarra, M J, Lannin, N A, Andrew, N & Reeder, S (2025). Relationship between staff experience and patient outcomes in hospital settings: an overview of reviews. *BMJ open*, *15*(1).
8   Avanzi, L, van Dick, R, Fraccaroli, F & Sarchielli, G (2012). The downside of organizational identification: Relations between identification, workaholism and wellbeing. *Work & Stress*, *26*(3), 289-307.
9   Maslach, C, Schaufeli, W B & Leiter, M P (2001). Job burnout. *Annual Review of Psychology*, *52*, 397-422.
10 For a review of the literature see Grawitch et al (2017). Creating a Psychologically Healthy Workplace p249-268 in Cooper & Leiter (eds) The Routledge Companion to Wellbeing at Work.
11 Maslach, C & Leiter, M P (2016). Understanding the burnout experience: recent research and its implications for psychiatry. *World Psychiatry: Official Journal of the World Psychiatric Association (WPA)*, *15*(2), 103-111.
12 The theory around culture is of course a bit more complex than this. For a review see:
13 Edmondson, A (1999). Psychological Safety and Learning Behaviour in Work Teams. *Administrative Science Quarterly*, *44*(2), 350-383.
14 Donohue, R (2017). 'Psychological safety: A systematic review of the literature', Human Resource Management Review.
15 de Lisser, R, Dietrich, M S, Spetz, J, Ramanujam, R, Lauderdale, J &

Stolldorf, D P (2024). Psychological safety is associated with better work environment and lower levels of clinician burnout. *Health Affairs Scholar*, 2(7).

16. Rasool, S F, Wang, M, Tang, M, Saeed, A & Iqbal, J (2021). How Toxic Workplace Environment Effects the Employee Engagement: The Mediating Role of Organizational Support and Employee Wellbeing. *International Journal of Environmental Research and Public Health*, 18(5), 2294.

17. Maslach C, Leiter M P. Early predictors of job burnout and engagement. J. Appl. Psychol. 2008;93:498–512.

18. Boddez, Y, Van Dessel, P & De Houwer, J (2022). Learned helplessness and its relevance for psychological suffering: a new perspective illustrated with attachment problems, burnout and fatigue complaints. *Cognition & Emotion*, 36(6), 1027–1036.

19. Laninga-Wijnen, L, Pouwels, J L, Giletta, M & Salmivalli, C (2024). Feeling better now? Being defended diminishes daily mood problems and self-blame in victims of bullying. *The British Journal of Educational Psychology*, 94(4), 1294–1322.

Chapter 7: Who cares? Caring and the other roles in our lives

1. Roskam, I & Mikolajczak, M (2023). Parental Burnout in the Context of Special Needs, Adoption and Single Parenthood. *Children (Basel, Switzerland)*, 10(7), 1131.

2. Mikolajczak, M, Gross, J J & Roskam, I (2021). Beyond Job Burnout: Parental Burnout! *Trends in Cognitive Sciences*, 25(5), 333–336. doi.org/10.1016/j.tics.2021.01.012
   Mikolajczak, M, Gross, J J, Stinglhamber, F, Lindahl, Norberg, A & Roskam, I (2020). Is parental burnout distinct from job burnout and depressive symptoms? *Clinical Psychological Science*, 8(4), 673–689. 10.1177/2167702620917447.
   Bornstein, M H (2020). 'Parental Burnout': The state of the science. *New Directions for Child and Adolescent Development*, 2020, 169–184. doi.org/10.1002/cad.20388

3. Roskam, I, Brianda, M-E & Mikolajczak, M (2018). A step forward in the conceptualization and measurement of parental burnout: The Parental Burnout Assessment (PBA). *Frontiers in Psychology*, 9, 758.

4. Mikolajczak, M, Gross, J J & Roskam, I (2019). Parental Burnout: What Is It, and Why Does It Matter? *Clinical Psychological Science*, 7(6), 1319–1329.

5. www.carersuk.org/media/rjknz2jt/state-of-caring-mental-health-and-social-care-feb-2025.pdf

Notes

6 www.carersuk.org/media/umaifzpq/cuk-state-of-caring-2024-finances-web.pdf
7 www.carersuk.org/media/rjknz2jt/state-of-caring-mental-health-and-social-care-feb-2025.pdf
8 www.som.org.uk/sites/som.org.uk/files/Burnout_in_healthcare_risk_factors_and_solutions_Jul23.pdf
9 www.bma.org.uk/media/2jhfvpgk/bma-covid-review-report-2-september-2024.pdf
Steven M A Bow, Peter Schröder-Bäck, Dominic Norcliffe-Brown, James Wilson, Farhang Tahzib, Moral distress and injury in the public health professional workforce during the COVID-19 pandemic, *Journal of Public Health*, Volume 45, Issue 3, September 2023, Pages 697–705.
10 committees.parliament.uk/publications/6158/documents/68766/default/
11 Baker, J & Vincent, R (2022). *The super-helper syndrome: a survival guide for compassionate people.* Flint Books.
12 wbg.org.uk/wp-content/uploads/2020/04/Accompanying-paper-FINAL.pdf
13 www.ons.gov.uk/employmentandlabourmarket/peopleinwork/earningsandworkinghours/articles/womenshouldertheresponsibilityofunpaidwork/2016-11-10
14 Dean, L, Churchill, B and Ruppanner, L (2021). The Mental Load: Building a Deeper Theoretical Understanding of How Cognitive and Emotional Labour Overload Women and Mothers. Community, Work and Family, 25(1), pp.13–29.
15 Daminger, A (2019). 'The Cognitive Dimension of Household Labour', American Sociological Review,84(4), pp.609–633.
16 Daminger, A (2019). How Couples Share 'Cognitive Labour' and Why it Matters. *Behavioural Scientist*.
17 Dean, L, Churchill, B & Ruppanner, L (2021). The Mental Load: Building a Deeper Theoretical Understanding of How Cognitive and Emotional Labour Overload Women and Mothers. Community, Work and Family, 25(1), pp.13–29.
18 Weeks, A C & Ruppanner, L (2025). A typology of US parents' mental loads: Core and episodic cognitive labour. *Journal of Marriage and Family*, 87(3), 966–989. doi.org/10.1111/jomf.13057
19 Beban, A & Roberts, G (2023). Fair but not Equal: Negotiating the Division of Unpaid Labour in Same-Sex Couples in Aotearoa New Zealand and Australia. *LGBTQ+ Family: An Interdisciplinary Journal*, 20(1), 74–91.

20 www.ons.gov.uk/employmentandlabourmarket/peopleinwork/earningsandworkinghours/articles/womenshouldertheresponsibility ofunpaidwork/2016-11-10
21 Dean, L, Churchill, B and Ruppanner, L (2021). The Mental Load: Building a Deeper Theoretical Understanding of How Cognitive and Emotional Labour Overload Women and Mothers. *Community, Work and Family*, 25(1), pp.13-29.
22 makemothersmatter.org/wp-content/uploads/2012/05/MMM-Report-Unpaid-cognitive-and-emotional-load-final.pdf
www.younglives.org.uk/publications/lightening-load-new-evidence-impacts-unpaid-care-work-women-and-girls
23 assets.publishing.service.gov.uk/media/653a577780884d000df71b86/WOW_Guidance_Note_on_Unpaid_care_and_domestic_work_PDF.pdf
24 Lakshmin, Pooja (2023). *Real Self-care: A Transformative Program for Redefining Wellness (Crystals, Cleanses and Bubble Baths Not Included)*. Penguin Life.
25 Thomas, S, Dalton, J, Harden, M, Eastwood, A & Parker, G (2017). *Updated meta-review of evidence on support for carers*. NIHR Journals Library. doi.org/10.3310/hsdr05120
26 Pratt, M (2024). *All in her head: how gender bias harms women's mental health*. Greystone Books.

Chapter 8: Different brains and burnout: Why burnout is a neurodiversity issue

1 Pugh, G E (1977). *The biological origin of human values*. Basic Book. In the book this quote is ascribed to his father, Emerson Pugh, also a physicist at MIT.
2 Zhang, F F, Peng, W, Sweeney, J A, Jia, Z Y & Gong, Q Y (2018). Brain structure alterations in depression: Psychoradiological evidence. *CNS Neuroscience & Therapeutics*, 24(11), 994-1003.
3 Chmiel, J & Malinowska, A (2025). Neural Correlates of Burnout Syndrome Based on Electroencephalography (EEG) - A Mechanistic Review and Discussion of Burnout Syndrome Cognitive Bias Theory. *Journal of Clinical Medicine*, 14(15), 5357.
4 Turjeman-Levi, Y, Itzchakov, G & Engel-Yeger, B (2024). Executive function deficits mediate the relationship between employees' ADHD and job burnout. *AIMS Public Health*, 11(1), 294-314.
Arnold, S R, Higgins, J M, Weise, J, Desai, A, Pellicano, E & Trollor, J N (2023). Towards the measurement of autistic burnout. *Autism: The International Journal of Research and Practice*, 27(7), 1933-1948.
Schatz, D B & Rostain, A L (2006). ADHD with comorbid anxiety: a

review of the current literature. *Journal of Attention Disorders*, *10*(2), 141-149.
5. Pellicano, E & den Houting, J (2022). Annual research review: Shifting from 'normal science' to neurodiversity in autism science. *Journal of Child Psychology and Psychiatry*, *63*(4), 381-396.
6. Botha, M & Frost, D M (2018). Extending the Minority Stress Model to Understand Mental Health Problems Experienced by the Autistic Population. *Society and Mental Health*, *10*(1), 20-34.
7. Oscarsson, M, Nelson, M, Rozental, A, Ginsberg, Y, Carlbring, P & Jönsson, F (2022). Stress and work-related mental illness among working adults with ADHD: a qualitative study. *BMC Psychiatry*, *22*(1), 751.
Combs, M A, Canu, W H, Broman-Fulks, J J, Rocheleau, C A & Nieman, D C (2012). Perceived Stress and ADHD Symptoms in Adults. *Journal of Attention Disorders*, *19*(5), 425-434.
Lin, L Y & Huang, P C (2017). Quality of life and its related factors for adults with autism spectrum disorder. *Disability and Rehabilitation*, *41*(8), 896-903.
8. Higgins, J M, Arnold, S R, Weise, J, Pellicano, E & Trollor, J N (2021). Defining autistic burnout through experts by lived experience: Grounded Delphi method investigating #AutisticBurnout. *Autism: The International Journal of Research and Practice*, *25*(8), 2356-2369.
9. Raymaker, D M, Teo, A R, Steckler, N A, Lentz, B, Scharer, M, Delos Santos, A, Kapp, S K, Hunter, M, Joyce, A & Nicolaidis, C (2020). 'Having All of Your Internal Resources Exhausted Beyond Measure and Being Left with No Clean-Up Crew': Defining Autistic Burnout. *Autism in Adulthood: Challenges and Management*, *2*(2), 132-143.
10. Miller, D, Rees, J & Pearson, A (2021). 'Masking Is Life': Experiences of Masking in Autistic and Nonautistic Adults. *Autism in Adulthood: Challenges and Management*, *3*(4), 330-338.
11. Higgins, J M, Arnold, S R, Weise, J, Pellicano, E & Trollor, J N (2021). Defining autistic burnout through experts by lived experience: Grounded Delphi method investigating #AutisticBurnout. *Autism: The International Journal of Research and Practice*, *25*(8), 2356-2369.
12. Mantzalas, J, Richdale, A L & Dissanayake, C (2022). A conceptual model of risk and protective factors for autistic burnout. *Autism Research: official journal of the International Society for Autism Research*, *15*(6), 976-987.
13. Arnold, S R, Higgins, J M, Weise, J, Desai, A, Pellicano, E & Trollor, J N (2023). Confirming the nature of autistic burnout. *Autism*, *27*(7), 1906-1918.
14. McQuaid, G A, Weiss, C H, Said, A J, Pelphrey, K A, Lee, N R & Wallace,

G L (2022). Perceived stress is negatively associated with activities of daily living and subjective quality of life in younger, middle and older autistic adults. *Autism Research*, 15, 1535-1549.

15 Kimber, L, Verrier, D & Connolly, S (2024). Autistic People's Experience of Empathy and the Autistic Empathy Deficit Narrative. *Autism in Adulthood: Challenges and Management*, 6(3), 321-330.

16 Shalev, I, Warrier, V, Greenberg, D M, Smith, P, Allison, C, Baron-Cohen, S, Eran, A & Uzefovsky, F (2022). Re-examining empathy in autism: Empathic disequilibrium as a novel predictor of autism diagnosis and autistic traits. *Autism Research: official journal of the International Society for Autism Research*, 15(10), 1917-1928.
www.bacp.co.uk/bacp-journals/bacp-workplace/2024/april/are-you-working-with-neurodivergent-burnout/

17 Huang, C, Wu, Z, Sha, S, Liu, C, Yang, L, Jiang, P, Zhang, H & Yang, C (2025). The Dark Side of Empathy: The Role of Excessive Affective Empathy in Mental Health Disorders. *Biological Psychiatry*, 98(5), 404-415.

18 Mantzalas, J, Richdale, A L & Dissanayake, C (2022). A conceptual model of risk and protective factors for autistic burnout. *Autism Research: official journal of the International Society for Autism Research*, 15(6), 976-987.

19 Shaw P, Stringaris A, Nigg J & Leibenluft E (2014). Emotion dysregulation in attention deficit hyperactivity disorder. Am J Psychiatry, 171(3): 276-293.
Mazefsky C A, Herrington J, Siegel M, Scarpa A, Maddox B B, Scahill L & White S W (2013). The role of emotion regulation in autism spectrum disorder. Journal of the American Academy of Child Adolescent Psychiatry; 52(7): 679-688.

20 Mantzalas, J, Richdale, A L, Li, X & Dissanayake, C (2024). Measuring and validating autistic burnout. *Autism research: official journal of the International Society for Autism Research*, 17(7), 1417-1449.

21 Niermann, H C & Scheres, A (2014). The relation between procrastination and symptoms of attention-deficit hyperactivity disorder (ADHD) in undergraduate students. *International Journal of Methods in Psychiatric Research*, 23(4), 411-421.

22 Ashinoff, B K & Abu-Akel, A (2021). Hyperfocus: the forgotten frontier of attention. *Psychological Research*, 85(1), 1-19.

23 Higgins, J M, Arnold, S R C, Weise, J, Smith, P, Pellicano, E & Trollor, J N (2021). Defining autistic burnout through experts by lived experience: Grounded Delphi method investigating #AutisticBurnout. *Autism*, 1-14, 2356-236.

24 Mantzalas, J, Richdale, A L & Dissanayake, C (2022). A conceptual model of risk and protective factors for autistic burnout. *Autism research: official journal of the International Society for Autism Research*, 15(6), 976-987.

Chapter 9: The emotional impact of burnout

1. May, K (2020). *Wintering: the power of rest and retreat in difficult times*. Rider.
2. Glise, K, Wiegner, L & Jonsdottir, I H (2020). Long-term follow-up of residual symptoms in patients treated for stress-related exhaustion. *BMC Psychol* 8, 26.
3. podcasts.apple.com/gb/podcast/mo-gawdat-part-1-looking-back-on-2020-the-year/id1508914142?i=1000503393251
4. Baumeister, R F, Bratslavsky, E, Finkenauer, C & Vohs, K D (2001). Bad is stronger than good. Review of General Psychology, 5(4), 323-370.
5. Khammissa, R A G, Nemutandani, S, Feller, G, Lemmer, J & Feller, L (2022). Burnout phenomenon: neurophysiological factors, clinical features and aspects of management. *The Journal of International Medical Research*, 50(9).

Chapter 10: The physical impact of burnout

1. For a summary of the research on the brain and body impact of burnout see:
Bayes, A, Tavella, G & Parker, G (2021). The biology of burnout: Causes and consequences. *The World Journal of Biological Psychiatry*, 22(9), 686-698.
Khammissa, R A G, Nemutandani, S, Feller, G, Lemmer, J & Feller, L (2022). Burnout phenomenon: neurophysiological factors, clinical features and aspects of management. *The Journal of International Medical Research*, 50(9).
van Dam, A (2021). A clinical perspective on burnout: diagnosis, classification and treatment of clinical burnout, European Journal of Work and Organizational Psychology, 30:5, 732-741.
Gavelin H M, Domellöf M E, Åström E, Nelson A, Launder N H, Neely A S, Lampit A. Cognitive function in clinical burnout: A systematic review and meta-analysis. Work Stress. 2021;36:86-104.
Some specific studies:
Chmiel, J & Malinowska, A (2025). Neural Correlates of Burnout Syndrome Based on Electroencephalography (EEG) - A Mechanistic Review and Discussion of Burnout Syndrome Cognitive Bias Theory. *Journal of Clinical Medicine*, 14(15), 5357.

Chmiel, J & Kurpas, D (2025). Burnout and the Brain – A Mechanistic Review of Magnetic Resonance Imaging (MRI) Studies. *International Journal of Molecular Sciences, 26*(17), 8379.

2 Bayes, A, Tavella, G & Parker, G (2021). The biology of burnout: Causes and consequences. *The World Journal of Biological Psychiatry, 22*(9), 686–698.

3 Bayes, A, Tavella, G & Parker, G (2021). The biology of burnout: Causes and consequences. *The World Journal of Biological Psychiatry, 22*(9), 686–698.

4 Khammissa, R A G, Nemutandani, S, Feller, G, Lemmer, J & Feller, L (2022). Burnout phenomenon: neurophysiological factors, clinical features and aspects of management. *The Journal of International Medical Research, 50*(9).
Nelson, A, Aronsson, I, Tillfors, M, Neely, A S & Gavelin, H M (2025). The experienced route to cognitive health: Cognitive recovery in persons with prior stress-related Exhaustion disorder. *BMC Psychiatry, 25*(1), 375.

5 Gannon, Emma. A Year of Nothing. (The Pound Project or HarperCollins, 2024 or 2025)

6 Gavelin H M, Domellöf M E, Åström E, Nelson A, Launder N H, Neely A S & Lampit, A. Cognitive function in clinical burnout: A systematic review and meta-analysis. Work Stress. 2021; 36:86–104.
Some specific studies:

7 Renaud, C & Lacroix, A (2023). Systematic review of occupational burnout in relation to cognitive functions: Current issues and treatments. International Journal of Stress Management, 30(2), 109–12.
Pihlaja, M, Tuominen, P P A, Peräkylä, J & Hartikainen, K M (2022). Occupational Burnout is Linked with Inefficient Executive Functioning, Elevated Average Heart Rate and Decreased Physical Activity in Daily Life – Initial Evidence from Teaching Professionals. *Brain Sciences, 12*(12), 1723.

8 Begeti, F (2024). *The Phone Fix: The Brain-Focused Guide to Building Healthy Digital Habits and Breaking Bad Ones*. Apollo: London.

9 lymphoma-action.org.uk/sites/default/files/media/documents/2020-05/Spoon%20theory%20by%20Christine%20Miserandino.pdf

Chapter 11: Piecing your life back together after burnout

1 www.bbc.co.uk/programmes/m0026x15
2 Hersey, T (2022). *Rest Is Resistance: A Manifesto*. First edition. Little, Brown Spark.
3 Dr Dalton-Smith (2018). *Sacred Rest: Renew your Energy, Restore your Sanity*. Faithwords.

Notes

4 Reading, S (2023). *Rest to Reset: The busy person's guide to pausing with purpose.* Octopus Publishing.
5 Burkeman, O (2025). *Meditation for Mortals: A Four Week Guide to Doing What Counts.* Vintage Publishing.

Chapter 12: Building back stronger

1 Galatzer-Levy, I R, Huang, S H & Bonanno, G A (2018). Trajectories of resilience and dysfunction following potential trauma: A review and statistical evaluation. *Clinical Psychology Review, 63,* 41-55.
2 www.bbc.co.uk/programmes/m0026x15
3 Dell'Osso, L, Lorenzi, P, Nardi, B, Carmassi, C & Carpita, B (2022). Post Traumatic Growth (PTG) in the Frame of Traumatic Experiences. *Clinical Neuropsychiatry, 19*(6), 390-393.
4 Frances, G (2022). *Recovery: The Lost Art of Convalescence.* Profile Books.
5 www.bbc.co.uk/programmes/m0026x15
6 Bronnie Ware (2012). *The Top Five Regrets of the Dying: A Life Transformed by the Dearly Departing.* Hay House Inc.
7 For a summary of the research in this area see: Lyubomjirsky, S (2014). *The Myths of Happiness.* Penguin.
8 Gannon, E (2024). *The Success Myth: Letting Go of Having It All.* Penguin.
9 donnalancaster.net
10 Hanel, P H P, Tunç, H, Bhasin, D, Litzellachner, L F & Maio, G R (2024). Value fulfilment and well-being: Clarifying directions over time. *Journal of Personality, 92*(4), 1037-1049.
11 Veage, S, Ciarrochi, J, Deane, F P, Andresen, R, Oades, L G & Crowe, T P (2014). Value congruence, importance and success and in the workplace: Links with well-being and burnout amongst mental health practitioners. *Journal of Contextual Behavioural Science,* 3, 258-264.

Acknowledgements

Thank you to everyone who helped me build this book. Kerry, Emily, Katie and the whole Quercus team, key book builders. Fraser, Evie and Stuart, my protective factors. Uta and Rona, early readers and negative ninja warriors. Susan and Rona, let's plan the next Edinburgh (or maybe further afield) trip.

Further Reading

My lens and other perspectives
Clinical Psychology recognizes that everyone's perspective is affected by their own lens, i.e. how they view the world based on their experiences. My lens is as a white Scottish female. In my clinical work, I have drawn across a range of people to help me share different perspectives and views; however, this is still filtered through my lens. Some authors who offer perspectives centred on different backgrounds include:

Radical Rest by Evie Muir; Elliott & Thompson, 2024
Women Who Work Too Much by Tamu Thomas; Hay House UK, 2024
Rest Is Resistance by Tricia Hersey; Aster, 2024
Black Fatigue: How racism erodes the mind, body and spirit by Mary-Frances Winters; Berrett-Koehler Publishers, 2020
Rest & Calm by Paula Hines; Green Tree, 2022
Decolonizing the Body by Christena Cleveland & Kelsey Blackwell; New Harbinger, 2023

Sleep
Bhutta, Z A, Bhavnani, S, Betancourt, T S et al. Adverse childhood experiences and lifelong health. Nat Med 29, 1639–1648 (2023).
McFarlane, A C (2010). The long-term costs of traumatic stress: intertwined physical and psychological consequences. World psychiatry: official journal of the World Psychiatric Association (WPA), 9(1), 3–10

Beliefs and burnout
How to Overcome Trauma and Find Yourself Again by Dr Jessamy Hibberd; Aster, 2024
The Art of Rest by Claudia Hammond; Canongate Books, 2020
How To Be Selfish by Suzy Reading; Vermilion, 2025
The Uncomfortable Truth by Anna Mathur; Penguin Life, 2024
The Success Myth by Emma Gannon; Penguin, 2024
Meditation for Mortals by Oliver Burkeman; Vintage, 2025
Four Thousand Weeks by Oliver Burkeman; Vintage, 2022
Can't Even: How millennials became the burnout generation by Anne Helen Petersen; Vintage, 2022
Saving Time: Discovering a life beyond the clock by Jenny Odell; Vintage, 2024
How To Do Nothing by Jenny Odell; Melville House Publishing, 2021

Further Reading

Sleep
Excellent overview of the functions of sleep: www.ninds.nih.gov/Disorders/Patient-Caregiver-Education/Understanding-Sleep

Stress
Roberts, B L & Karatsoreos, I N (2021). Brain-body responses to chronic stress: a brief review. Faculty reviews, 10, 83
Schneiderman, N, Ironson, G & Siegel, S D (2005). Stress and health: psychological, behavioural and biological determinants. Annual review of clinical psychology, 1, 607–628. doi.org/10.1146/annurev.clinpsy.1.102803.144141

Creating anti-burnout workplaces
Reworked by Dr Stephanie Fitzgerald; John Murray Business, 2023
Coaching Through Burnout by Hazel Anderson-Turner; The Unbound Press, 2025
How To Work Without Losing Your Mind by Cate Sevilla; Penguin, 2023
You Coach You by Helen Tupper & Sarah Ellis; Penguin Business, 2022

Tackling the mental load
Fair Play: Share the mental load, rebalance your relationship and change your life by Eve Rodksy; Quercus, 2021
The Fair Play Deck
A Better Share: How couples can tackle the mental load for more fun, less resentment and great sex by Dr Morgan Cutlip; Thomas Nelson, 2025

Neurodivergence and burnout
Neurodiversity for Dummies by John Marble, Khushboo Chabria & Ranga Jayaraman; For Dummies, 2024
Explaining AuDHD by Khurram Sadiq; August Books, 2025
The Autistic Burnout Workbook: Your guide to your personal recovery plan (self-care for autistic people) by Dr Megan Anna Neff; Adams Media, 2025
Unmasking for Life by Dr Devon Price; Monoray, 2025
The Autistic Brain by Temple Grandin & Richard Panek; Rider, 2014
Untypical: How the world isn't built for autistic people and what we should all do about it by Pete Wharmby; Mudlark, 2024
It's Not a Bloody Trend: Understanding life as an ADHD adult by Kat Brown; Robinson, 2025
Is It My ADHD? by Grace Timothy; Allen & Unwin, 2025
How to ADHD by Jessica McCabe; Souvenir Press, 2024

The Anti-Burnout Book

Dirty Laundry: Why adults with ADHD are so ashamed and what we can do to help by Richard Pink & Roxanne Emery; Square Peg, 2023

Softening shame
Emma Gannon's Substack: thehyphen.substack.com
www.audible.co.uk/podcast/Parental-Burnout-Is-Real-You-Cant-Pour-From-an-Empty-Cup-with-Lisa-Galley/B0F9W1N3YB
Illuminated, In Pieces www.bbc.co.uk/programmes/m0026x15
How to Keep House While Drowning by K C Davis; Penguin, 2024
I Thought It Was Just Me by Brené Brown; Penguin, 2007
Daring Greatly by Brené Brown; Penguin, 2015

Cutting back and creating space
Joy of Saying No by Natalie Lue; Harper Christian Resources, 2023
Set Boundaries, Find Peace by Nedra Glover Tawwab; Piatkus, 2021
A Year of Nothing by Emma Gannon; Whitefox Publishing Ltd, 2026

Validating experiences
Burnout by Emily & Amelia Nagoski; Vermilion, 2020
All in her Head by Misty Pratt; Greystone Books, 2025

Self-compassion
Mindful Self-compassion for Burnout by Kirsten Neff, Christopher Germer & Christine M. Benton; Guilford Press, 2024
Mindful Compassion by Paul Gilbert; Robinson, 2015

Learning to rest
Rest to Reset by Suzy Reading; Aster, 2023
The Art of Rest by Claudia Hammond; Canongate Books, 2020
The Nap Ministry's Rest Deck

Looking at your values
Information on values: thehappinesstrap.com/category/values/
Working out your values worksheet: thehappinesstrap.com/upimages/Values_Questionnaire.pdf\
List of values: www.actmindfully.com.au/wp-content/uploads/2019/07/Values_Checklist_-_Russ_Harris.pdf
Values reflection toolkit: reflection.ed.ac.uk/reflectors-toolkit/self-awareness/values
Values worksheet: brenebrown.com/resources/living-into-our-values/

Index

achievement 97-9, 100, 109, 121
ADHD 170-1, 174
adrenaline 72
alertness, hyper- 18
amygdala 71, 213
anxiety 30, 73, 180
attention 63, 74, 182-3, 222
autistic burnout 174-5, 183
autonomic nervous system 71, 74
awareness 266-8
awe, recapturing 248-9

background factors 48-9
Begeti, Dr Faye 222
behaviours 50-1, 91, 137
beliefs 50, 85-105
   about emotions 110, 111-12
   belief-shifting 88-9
   building your own manifesto 104
   how belief systems impact life 88
   how beliefs build in our brain 86-8
   how we view ourselves 99-100, 102
   identifying unhelpful beliefs 93-4
   influences on 87, 89
   mythical land of THERE 94-6, 101, 146
   productivity, achievement and rest 97-9
   societal beliefs 172-3
   toxic work cultures and 133
   undoing the messaging 102-4
   what beliefs are 86-91
bias 88
   negative 18-19, 90-1, 206

   unconscious bias 89, 92
blame: blame cultures 135-6
   self-blame 38-40, 142, 177, 214, 224
the body: the body and burnout 213-15
   physical and emotional needs 106-19
   why we battle our body signals 108-10
body budget 106-7, 111
   bringing it out of debt 218-20
   and burnout 113-16
   managing 114-16
   parental burnout 147
bouncing back 201-3
boundaries 280-1
the brain 89, 213-15
   brain factors, environmental interactions and burnout 176-83
   burnout and brain function 169-70
   burnout as a neurodiversity issue 166-87
   chronic stress 73-5
   cognitive functioning 168-9, 170, 176, 221-2, 223
   helpful body stress response 70-3
   how beliefs build in our brain 86-8, 103
   interoception and the body budget 106-7
   low power mode 221-4, 226, 258, 259

negative bias 18-19, 90-1
stress body response 66
your brain and burnout exercise
   184-6
breaks 140
Burkeman, Oliver 254
burnout: burnout scale 33-4
  burnout tree 41-60, 132, 147,
    160, 190-1
  definition of 14-16
  how to avoid 61-187
  physical impact of 212-34
  physical pathways out of 215-34
  recovering from 235-61
  symptoms 17-24, 267-8
  what to do if you are burned out
    188-289

capacity: boosting your capacity
   162-3
  capacity cup 66-9, 147, 156, 163,
    180
  capacity overflow and overwhelm
    227-30
  working with minimal capacity
    227
care roles 144-65
  caring as a profession 149-50,
    152
  caring for the world 151-2
  caring for yourself with illness or
    a disability 151
  cost of caring 153
  motherhood juggle 145-6
  other unpaid care roles 148-9
  parental burnout 146-8
  super helpers 150, 152
  systems around caring roles and
    burnout 160-4
change 142, 285-7
characteristics 50

children and childhood: beliefs and
   87, 89
  difficult childhoods 49
  motherhood juggle 145-6
  parental burnout 146-8
clarity 140
cognition 215
  cognitive empathy 179
  cognitive functioning 168-9, 170,
    176, 221-2, 223
  cognitive load 155, 178-9, 224
community 130, 141
compassion 200, 209, 248
  compassion fatigue 152
  self-compassion 204, 284-5
connections, social 284
context factors 41, 44, 53
control 129, 141, 236
  regaining 253-4
  relinquishing 255-7
coping styles 50
cortisol 72, 74, 213
criticism, inner 203-5, 213-14, 228,
    235, 248
cultures: characteristics of work
    cultures 53-4
  general work cultures 130-2
  not buying into culture edicts 140
  toxic work cultures 127, 131,
    133-6
Currie, Lauren 103-4
cynicism, work related 16, 18-19

Dalton-Smith, Dr 251
depersonalizing work 141-2
depression 30-1, 168
digestive issues 73, 74
disability, caring for yourself with
    151
discrimination 177-8
distractibility 183

Index

domestic labour 155-6, 157

Edmondson, Amy 130
efficacy, reduced personal 16, 20
effort 178-9
elderly, caring for 148
emotions 281
  and body budget 113-16
  difficult emotions 209-10
  emotion processing 180-1
  emotional empathy 179
  emotional impact of burnout 190-211
  emotional load 155
  emotional needs 106-19
  emotional pathways out of burnout 192-210
  emotions as body signals 110-12, 117, 118
  emotions as data 116-19
  feel-good emotions 248
  suppressing 109
empathy 152, 179
energy 281
  depletion of 16, 17
  energy levels at work 140
  low power mode 221-4, 226, 258, 259
  protecting and managing 231-3
  spoon theory 232-3
  things that replenish 251
environment: changing your 285-7
  environmental interactions and burnout 176-83
executive functioning factors 181-2, 221, 222
exhaustion 16, 17, 235
expectations, shifting your 225-6
experiences, legitimizing 192-5
eyes, twitching 62, 75

the 'F it!' bucket 282
fairness 130
fatigue 29, 152
Feldman-Barrett, Lisa 107
fight or flight response 72-3, 213, 228
focused attention 182
Francis, Dr Gavin 263-4
Freudenberger, H J 15

Gannon, Emma 19, 215-16, 269
Gawdat, Mo 203
gender 48
Gilbert, Elizabeth 284-5
Great Big Blazing Burnout Quiz 46-59
guilt 147, 150, 164, 277

habits, replacing harmful 258-60
hair loss 62-3, 75
health 48
  effect of stress on 66, 74-5
helplessness 133-4
Hersey, Tricia 250
Higgens, J M 174
home life 27-8
  care and other roles in your life 144-65
  work-life balance 37-8, 131, 139
homeostasis 71
hope, holding on to 195-7
hyperactivity 183
hyper-alertness 18
hypothalamus 71

identity 138, 236
  rebuilding your 243-5
  work and 123-5
illness 29, 151
immune system 74-5, 213
impulsivity 182

inner critics 213-14, 228, 235, 248
  don't be a sh*t to yourself 203-5
  transforming your 205
internal causal attribution 135-6

joy, recapturing 248-9

knowledge 266-8

Lakshmin, Dr Pooja 160
legitimizing experiences 192-5
life 27-8
  care and other roles in your life 144-65
  life impact of burnout 235-8
  life stages 47
  work-life balance 37-8, 131, 139

masking 176-7
Maslach, C 15, 16, 25
Maslach Burnout Inventory 21
May, Katherine 20, 191
memory 63, 74, 222
mental flexibility 181
mental health 28-32, 66, 100, 121-2
mental load 153-9
messiness, embracing 253-5
Miserandino, Christine 232
mothers: mental load 153-9
  motherhood juggle 145-6
  parental burnout 146-8

needs, understanding your 240-2
negativity 88
  internalizing a negative culture 135-6
  negative bias 18-19, 90-1, 206
  negative ninjas 206-9, 213-14, 248
  view of ourselves 99-100, 102
  work related 16, 18-19

nervous system 71-2, 73, 74, 80
neurodiversity 48, 166-87
  helping a neurodivergent brain be anti-burnout 183-4
  neurodivergent burnout 174-86
  and our idea of neurotypical 172
'no', saying 277-80
non-negotiables, committing to your 275-7

ocular myokymia 62, 75
opening up 103
organizing 181-2
overwhelm 66, 77, 148, 156
  capacity overflow and 227-30
  six steps to stopping 229-30

parasympathetic nervous system 71, 74, 80
parents: caring for elderly 148
  motherhood juggle 145-6
  parental burnout 146-8
pathways out of burnout 215-34
perfection 100, 101, 128, 284
perpetuating factors 41, 42
personal factors 137, 138
perspective disconnect 177
physical health, impact of burnout 212-34
physical needs 106-19
planning 181-2
powering on 250
Pratt, Misty 161
prefrontal cortex 213, 221
pressure 62-84, 93, 283
productivity 97-9, 109, 138, 245
protective factors 41, 42, 51
Pugh, George 167

Reading, Suzy 251
reconnecting 246-7

Index

recovery 262-88
   the art of recovery 263-4
   creating space for 215-18
reductions, using to grow 283-5
reflection 138
resilience 138, 201
resources, protecting your precious 280-1
rest 97-9, 103, 193, 249-53, 276
   learning to rest 251-3, 255-8
rest and digest system 74, 80-3
reward 129
rights 142
risk factors 41, 42, 50-1
roots, regrowing 246-7

Schaffner, Anna Katharina 97-8
self-preservation society 277-82
Selye, Hans 64
sensory processing sensitivity 180
shame 142, 223, 228, 235
   about burnout 38, 39, 40-1, 132
   about emotions 112
   negativity bias 90, 103
   neurodiversity and 184
   saying 'hello' and 'goodbye' to shame 212-13
   softening your shame 198-201
sleep 49, 77, 276
slowing down 283
social connections 284
solutions, suggesting 141
space, creating for recovery 215-18
spoon theory 232-3
stigma 176, 177-8
stress 62-84
   antidotes to 80-3
   awareness of factors that contribute to 176
   benefits of 63, 66
   chronic stress 66, 73-6

coping strategies 77-8
   cumulative 37
   definition of 64-9
   exponential growth of the stress weed 76-80
   fertilizing the stress weed 77-80
   helpful body stress response 70-3
   levels of 66
   managing stress levels 67-9
   and negative bias 206
   and societal beliefs 173
   spotting the signs of toxic stress 75-6
   stress body response 66, 80
   stress weed suppression and prevention 79-80
   symptoms of 62-3
   when stress becomes unhelpful 70-80
   and work 16, 122, 125-7
stressors 42, 52-3, 63, 64, 65
   fight or flight response 73
   neurodiversity and 178
   thoughts as 85
   work 123, 133
success, redefining your metrics of 268-70
super helpers 150, 152
support 141, 142
   accepting 285
   neurodiversity and 178
Swift, Taylor 231
switching off 139
sympathetic nervous system 71-2, 73, 80
symptoms, recognising 267-8
systemic factors 41, 44, 54-5, 137, 138, 141-2

talking things through 141

therapy 194
THERE, mythical land of 94-6, 101, 146
thoughts 85-6
time pressures 283
tiny thing tsunami 163-4
toxic work culture 131, 133-6
trauma 49, 65, 102, 149-50

unconscious bias 89, 92
understanding 195

validation 194
value, work-related 129
values 271-4, 281

Walker-Brown, Hannah 240, 265
wants, understanding your 240-2
Ware, Bronnie 265
wellbeing 121, 122-5, 128-30, 201
willpower 258, 259, 260
women: caring roles 153-4
   domestic labour 26-7, 145-6, 155-6
   mental load 153-9
   motherhood juggle 145-6
wonder, recapturing 248-9
work: burnout-creating systems 128-30
   career stage 48
   characteristics of the culture 53-4
   characteristics of the people around you 54
   characteristics of your role 53
   definition of in the modern world 26-7
   general culture 130-2
   how you feel at work 126-7
   jobs as part of our identity 98
   locating where the issues exist 138-41
   making work work for you 120-43
   negativity related to 16, 18-19, 49
   and stress 16, 25-7, 122, 125-7
   toxic work culture 127, 131, 133-6
   type of job 47
   unpaid work 26-7, 145-6, 155-6
   ups and downs of working life 121-2
   when to leave work 142
   work and identity 123-5
   work/life balance 37-8, 131, 139
   work, wellbeing and burnout 122-5
   workplace systems and burnout 127-36, 140
World Health Organization (WHO) 15, 16, 25, 30
worth 100

'yes', saying 277-80

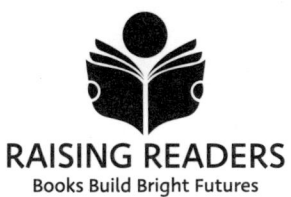

RAISING READERS
Books Build Bright Futures

Dear Reader,

We'd love your attention for one more page to tell you about the crisis in children's reading, and what we can all do.

Studies have shown that reading for fun is the **single biggest predictor of a child's future life chances** – more than family circumstance, parents' educational background or income. It improves academic results, mental health, wealth, communication skills, ambition and happiness.[1]

The number of children reading for fun is in rapid decline. Young people have a lot of competition for their time. In 2024, 1 in 10 children and young people in the UK aged 5 to 18 did not own a single book at home.[2]

Hachette works extensively with schools, libraries and literacy charities, but here are some ways we can all raise more readers:

- Reading to children for just 10 minutes a day makes a difference
- Don't give up if children aren't regular readers – there will be books for them!
- Visit bookshops and libraries to get recommendations
- Encourage them to listen to audiobooks
- Support school libraries
- Give books as gifts

There's a lot more information about how to encourage children to read on our website: **www.RaisingReaders.co.uk**

Thank you for reading.

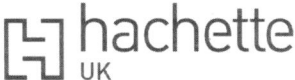

---

[1] OECD, '21st-Century Readers: Developing Literacy Skills in a Digital World', 2021, https://www.oecd.org/en/publications/21st-century-readers_a83d84cb-en.html

[2] National Literacy Trust, 'Book Ownership in 2024', November 2024, https://literacytrust.org.uk/research-services/research-reports/book-ownership-in-2024

First published in Great Britain in 2026 by Greenfinch
An imprint of Quercus
Part of John Murray Group

Text and illustration copyright © 2026 Dr Emma Hepburn

The moral right of Dr Emma Hepburn to be identified as the author of this work has beenasserted in accordance with the Copyright, Designs and Patents Act, 1988.

All rights reserved. No part of this publication may be reproduced or transmitted in any form or by any means, electronic or mechanical, including photocopy, recording, or any information storage and retrieval system, without permission in writing from the publisher.

A CIP catalogue record for this book is available from the British Library

HB ISBN 978-1-52944-544-2
TPB ISBN 978-1-52944-545-9
EBOOK ISBN 978-1-52944-546-6

10 9 8 7 6 5 4 3 2 1

Quercus hereby exclude all liability to the extent permitted by law for any errors or omissions in this book and for any loss, damage or expense (whether direct or indirect) suffered by a third party relying on any information contained in this book.

Typeset by seagulls.net
Cover design by Steve Leard
Printed and bound in Great Britain by Clays Ltd, Elcograf S.p.A.

Papers used by Quercus are from well-managed forests and other responsible sources.

Quercus
Carmelite House
50 Victoria Embankment
London EC4Y 0DZ

John Murray Group
Part of Hodder & Stoughton Limited
An Hachette UK company

The authorised representative in the EEA is Hachette Ireland, 8 Castlecourt Centre, Dublin 15, D15 XTP3, Ireland (email: info@hbgi.ie)